Bicycling

CLIMB!

Bicycling

CLIMB!

CONQUER HILLS, GET LEAN, AND ELEVATE EVERY RIDE

SELENE YEAGER AND THE EDITORS OF BICYCLING

HEARST

The information in this book is meant to supplement, not replace, proper exercise training. All forms of exercise pose some inherent risks. The editors and publisher advise readers to take full responsibility for their safety and know their limits. Before practicing the exercises in this book, be sure that your equipment is well-maintained, and do not take risks beyond your level of experience, aptitude, training, and fitness. The exercise and dietary programs in this book are not intended as a substitute for any exercise routine or dietary regimen that may have been prescribed by your doctor. As with all exercise and dietary programs, you should get your doctor's approval before beginning.

Mention of specific companies, organizations, or authorities in this book does not imply endorsement by the author or publisher, nor does mention of specific companies, organizations, or authorities imply that they endorse this book, its author, or the publisher.

Internet addresses and phone numbers given in this book were accurate at the time it went to press.

© 2018 by Hearst Magazines, Inc.

All rights reserved. No part of this publication may be reproduced or transmitted in any form or by any means, electronic or mechanical, including photocopying, recording, or any other information storage and retrieval system, without the written permission of the publisher.

Bicycling® is a registered trademark of Hearst Magazines, Inc.

Printed in the United States of America

Cover photo by Stephen Fleming/Alamy Stock Photo
Interior photos by Mitch Mandel

Book design by Tim Solliday, Jordan Wannemacher, and Cindy Webster

Library of Congress Cataloging-in-Publication Data is on file with the publisher.

ISBN 978-1-950099-42-9

9   10   11   paperback

HEARST

To my friends, family, and everyone who has helped me climb,
both on and off the bike.

CONTENTS

ACKNOWLEDGMENTS — ix
INTRODUCTION: WHY YOU SHOULD CLIMB — xi

1. HIGH TIDES — 1
2. PHYSICS — 13
3. GOATS AND GRINDERS — 23
4. BASE CAMP — 37
5. YOUR POWER STATION — 57
6. F%CK! — 75
7. WHEELS IN THE SKY — 89
8. WEIGHTY MATTERS — 99
9. WHAT GOES UP . . . — 115

10. SMALL BUT MIGHTY 125
11. THERE BE MONSTERS 141
12. PULLING IT ALL TOGETHER:
TRAINING PLANS AND CLIMBING CHALLENGES 157

    REFERENCES 185
    INDEX 189

ACKNOWLEDGMENTS

▶ **NO ONE MAKES IT** up the big mountains alone. It takes a team of planners, supporters, and executors, and I have had a dream team to make it up the mountain of writing this book. I'd like to thank my editors and colleagues at *Bicycling* who have helped lift me along on this editorial climb from notion to execution, especially Bill Strickland, Leah Flickinger, Emily Furia, Kris Siessmayer, Mitch Mandel, Tim Solliday, Amy King, Alisa Bowman, Marilyn Hauptly, Sara Cox, Shannon Mushock, and Lisa Andruscavage. You've made this project a great ride.

INTRODUCTION
Why You Should Climb

▶ **REVELATIONS RARELY COME AS** light bulbs, the way they're shown in cartoons—popping up in a bubble during someone's most vexing moments. But, this one did. It was my first major mountain bike race—the 24 Hours of Canaan—and I was a bundle of hypoxic nerves, legs searing like blackened steaks up what seemed like an eternal climb. I started to wonder if, somewhere at the top of one of these monsters in West-by-God Virginia, I might actually meet my maker, when I turned a corner onto the hardest, longest climb of the course—a seemingly endless series of switchbacks that would eventually emerge at the bottom of Canaan Valley Resort's Salamander Slope, what my fellow racers simply called the wall.

Light was dimming as the sun started to set, darkening my mood as it sank behind the distant rolling ranges. Head down, I churned along the gravel road with a growing sense of gloom—I would have two, maybe three more trips up this monster. I glanced to the roadside at my left, where a tan, lean, long-limbed local was fixing a flat and smoking some weed. "Hey!" he called out to me as I turned my head back to the task at hand. I glanced back. He flashed a sincere smile that lit up his face from his glassy eyes to his bearded chin. "Enjoy the climb. It's a beautiful one!"

I shook my head, but somewhere deep inside the recesses of my mind, I flipped a switch. I turned my eyes from the gravel and mud of the ground beneath my tires to the rolling misty mountains kissed with orange and pink surrounding me. It *was* really beautiful. Sure, it was hard. But, that didn't mean I couldn't enjoy it, embrace it, hell, even double-down and challenge it right back. I shifted gears, stood on my pedals, and actually smiled for the first time since leaving the starting gate. And, though I suffered dearly up Salamander and its 20-plus percent finishing grade, I sincerely enjoyed that mother. And, in one way or another, either during or after the fact (and yes, more than a few *far after* the facts), I've enjoyed every hill, mountain, roller, and wall since.

Climbing, I've come to learn, is more than a physical task. The act of pedaling your bike to the peak of a distant bump on the horizon is transformative. Years after that West Virginia awakening, I remember sitting outside the mess tent at the ABSA Cape Epic stage race in Oak Valley, South Africa, watching the sun rise over the majestic and somewhat ominous Hottentots Holland Mountains and laughing out loud at the realization that I was going to take my little white mountain bike and pedal up and over those sky-kissing summits from the shores of the Atlantic to the coast of the Indian Ocean. At the end of the day, I spontaneously burst into tears when I spied that vast shimmering body of water in the distance. The day had been brutally hot. The terrain, ungroomed and unforgiving. My back ached, my legs burned, I drifted back and forth over the border of bonking. Today, I remember it all with nothing but fondness, and I have found myself on those mountains in my mind's eye many times when faced with adversity that seems insurmountable. Because those mountains taught me better.

That is why I encourage everyone who will listen to climb as much as they can and why I have made it much of my life's work to learn as much about climbing as possible. The rewards are immediate, lasting, and transcendent.

Climb! is the culmination of 20 years of studying, training, racing, coaching, interviewing, absorbing, seemingly endless rambling and ruminating, and ultimately accumulating all the climbing know-how I could.

It's all in here: Everything you need to know to make meaningful and measurable improvements in your climbing, including the physics of riding uphill; the muscles and fuel you use when you're fighting the forces of gravity; how to apply the right gearing (and how to use the gears you have); how to fuel, train, and recover for long days filled with lots of elevation; how to get past negative self-talk and propel yourself with positivity; how to position yourself in (and out of) the saddle and pick the right cadence for maximum power and efficiency for shallow as well as steep grades; how to strengthen your key climbing muscles off the bike; what power-to-weight ratio really means; and so many intangibles that add to the success—and the joy—of the ascent.

But *Climb!* is much more than a how-to guide. It's a celebration of some of the world's most storied ascents and some of the best stories from those who have experienced them from behind the handlebars of a bike. I'm psyched to share it all right here. Let's take it to and from the top.

1 | HIGH TIDES

The more you climb, the greater the rewards—on and off the bike.

▶ **THE FIRST TIME** T. J. Klausutis laid eyes on Saint Kevin's, a steep, 4.3-mile two-track, gravel road that marks the first massive challenge on the 104-mile Leadville mountain bike racecourse in Colorado, he was 275 pounds . . . and had been training on the flapjack-flat Florida panhandle. "It firmly planted a foot up my ass . . . it was an awakening," he recalls. The awakenings would only get ruder.

Next up was Sugarloaf Pass, a sustained climb that comes 13 miles into the day. T. J. was determined to attack, because that's what he did in Florida when he and his training mates hit climbs. They attacked to get them over with. The problem is that Sugarloaf is 5 miles long. "Forget the weight issue for a moment; I just didn't know what I was doing," he says. He overheated and had to walk to cool down—but got back on his bike and kept going.

Then, came Columbine—an 8-mile, 3,200-foot climb, which starts deceptively easily on smooth pavement and easy grades but ever so slowly transforms into a rocky goat path hellscape that tops out at 12,600 feet of elevation at the Columbine Mine. "Again, I figured I would just spin and get it over with. I couldn't conceive how long it was, and, because the first part is tree-lined, you can't really see how long it is . . . I blew myself up and was off the bike within a mile, alternating between pushing and pedaling. Once I got to the rocky part, I was stumbling and could barely even push my bike."

He made it up Columbine, but he'd burned too many matches to be able to finish the event. He was pulled off-course at mile 60 for missing the time cut by a heartbreaking 14 seconds. "I'd come completely unprepared."

Beaten down, but not out, T. J. was determined to return to those mountains and emerge victorious (which at Leadville means completing the course in under 12 hours, earning you a nice shiny belt buckle as a reward). The learning curve, however, proved as steep as those monstrous mountains of the Colorado Rockies. He came back the following year, better trained, but still 275 pounds and still not quite mentally ready for the challenge. This time, he made it two-thirds of the way up Pipeline, a long, rutted, blustery pass about three-quarters of the way through the event, before missing a time cut and being pulled a second time.

Furious with himself, but determined to get it right, T. J., with the help of his girlfriend, buckled down and "trained his weakness"—climbing. "We did a mix of 'Florida tricks,' because you need to be creative when there aren't many hills to train on," he says. "We went out and did hard rides into headwinds and took some trips to Alabama to do hill repeats in Oak Mountain State Park."

T. J. also worked on his diet: He started eating more protein and healthy fat and limiting starchy carbs when he wasn't on his bike. He also set his mind to embrace the suck. "I accepted that it's going to suck, because it's supposed to. Don't panic because it hurts. It's supposed to hurt! You just settle in, and embrace the pain. The suffering means that you're doing it right."

The next time he lined up at Leadville, he was 220 pounds—still a big man on a bike, but more than 50 pounds lighter—and more determined than ever. He still had to walk a few times, but he settled in, stayed calm, and worked his way up each and every incline on that 104-mile course. He finished in 11:36, finally earning that coveted buckle.

YOUR BEST FRENEMIES (WITH BENEFITS)

Though some riders learn to love (or always have loved) climbs, for riders like T. J., it's a bit more of a love-hate relationship, frenemies with benefits, if you will. "I do not love climbing!" he says emphatically. "I am proud that I have the ability to do it. And, it's amazing to look back after making a climb and realizing that I can do this now. It is also really fun to surprise people. I have heard more cheers for the big guy! It is not love, but it's a hell of a sense of accomplishment, which transcends the bike."

It's like the old saying "a rising tide lifts all boats." Overcoming the hurdles that kept him from climbing not only made T. J. leaner, stronger, smarter, more skilled, and mentally tougher on the bike, but also it gave him the confidence to keep pushing himself. He's since collected four more of those shiny Leadville buckles and taken on other massive cycling challenges, like the Dirty Kanza 200 (a grueling 200-mile gravel event in the Flint Hills region of Kansas) and the infamous La Ruta de los Conquistadores (a race in Costa Rica, which climbs 25,344 feet in 3 days!). He also has plans to compete in a full-length Ironman Triathlon.

But, what makes climbing so transformative? Let's take a closer look.

THE METABOLIC MAGIC

When you tackle an ascent, adaptations happen inside every cell of your body. Whether you're a large flatlander like T. J., a natural mountain goat, or anything in between, as the road tilts up, your body undergoes a cascade of reactions that may kind of hurt in the moment but are oh-so-good for you in the long term. Here's what's happening to your body on a climb.

YOUR LEGS: Your average 15-minute climb is the equivalent of doing 1,200 little leg presses to the top. That makes hills as good as gold, or I should say Gold's, for building strength. It's simple physics (which you'll learn more about in the next chapter). As you pedal up a grade, gravity tries to pull you back down. The steeper the pitch, the more forceful gravity's pull. This means that you need to recruit more muscles to maintain forward momentum. Climbing hills—especially seated climbing—engages your glutes, quads, and calves to a larger degree than when you are spinning along the flats. Climbing not only builds neuromuscular connections—so you have more muscle fibers turned on and at your disposal—but also breaks down the small fibers in your muscles, which rebuild stronger when you rest, making that same monster climb a little easier over time.

YOUR HEART: With more muscles being called to action, your heart has to work harder to supply oxygen and nutrient-rich blood where it's needed. All that effort also creates heat, which means more work for your heart, as it needs to send blood to your skin to help you sweat and keep cool. The result: Your heart rate will be 30 to 40 bpm higher when you're cranking up a hill than when you're cruising along level ground. Standing and climbing out of the saddle drives up your heart rate 5 to 10 beats further because you're engaging your upper body in the movement, and those arms, shoulders, and back muscles need to consume more oxygen. All of this effort makes your heart stronger, so it can squeeze out more blood with every beat. This is why fit cyclists have resting heart rates 10 to 15 beats lower than their unconditioned peers.

YOUR CIRCULATORY SYSTEM: It does you no good for your heart to be pumping out blood like an open fire hydrant if your body can't deliver all that essential fluid into the muscles that need it. Climbing hills increases demands on your blood delivery system, so your body responds by forging more capillaries into your muscles. This lets your muscle cells have all the blood they need to get ample amounts of oxygen and nutrients to produce energy.

YOUR MITOCHONDRIA: Your energy demands spike along with the ride profile, so your cells' energy-producing furnaces—the mitochondria—go into overdrive to deliver all the oxygen and fuel your muscles need to do their work. Your body adapts by multiplying and building up your existing mitochondria, which helps you use oxygen more effectively as well as process lactate (an essential muscle fuel source). That's why climbing hills helps raise your lactate threshold (the point at which you cross over from low- to high-intensity exercise), which, in turn, allows you to stay aerobic and burn fat at higher effort levels. That means that you can ride faster, harder, and longer before fatiguing.

YOUR LUNGS: All the oxygen being used by your energy-producing mitochondria has to come from somewhere, and that somewhere is your respiratory system. As your heart rate goes up and your stroke volume increases, there's more blood pouring through your lungs. You not only breathe faster but also you breathe more deeply to expand and enlarge your alveoli (the grapelike sacs where oxygen is exchanged for carbon dioxide), so you get more oxygen with every breath.

YOUR CORE: Climbing requires so much core work that racers like multi-time world champion mountain bike racer Rebecca Rusch, who once rode her bike up Mount Kilimanjaro, the highest peak in Africa (which kisses the sky at 19,341 feet), use uphill efforts as part of their core-strengthening routine. For one, you use your core muscles to maintain a solid platform for your legs to work against as your cadence slows and your effort increases. Your abs, back, and sides are also your power transfer center, as the force you generate pulling the bars transfers through your core and is transmitted into your lower body to increase the force that you can apply to your pedals. Those anchor muscles engage even more to stabilize you when you get out of the saddle to climb.

That laborious effort extends all the way into your deepest core muscles as you draw in and push out hard, deep breaths. Pulmonary expert Paul W. Davenport, PhD, of the Center for Respiratory Research and Rehabilitation at the University of Florida likens it to the effort required to pump up your tires. It's a breeze to inflate them to the lower end of their recommended psi range, but as you approach the upper limits, it takes more force to pump in each pound. The same is true for your internal airbags. "Normally, you sit at a baseline midpoint, where you still have some air in your lungs—your expiratory reserve—when you exhale," says Dr. Davenport. When you're exercising, especially doing something hard like hill climbing, you use part of that expiratory reserve and blow out more than you would at rest. To assist, your body recruits muscles—primarily your abdominals and diaphragm—to blow out more air faster, so you can get more in faster.

YOUR BRAIN: Climbing is as much mental training as it is physical. (That's why the better chunk of Chapter 6 covers the territory between your ears, including brain-training techniques such as self-talk, visualization, and focus.) What's fascinating is that not only do your thoughts shape how you climb but also your climbing alters your thoughts—on and off the bike—via hormonal changes that happen inside your gray matter when you head uphill.

It comes down to the suffering. Like T. J. says, hills are hard. Pedaling up and over them, even if it's what you call fun, is a form of stress—healthy stress, but stress nonetheless. Your body responds to that stress by releasing cortisol to raise your heart rate, blood pressure, and blood glucose levels. As you get fitter, it takes a longer, harder ride—i.e., hills—to trigger that same response. But, there's a payoff. You can handle more stress without wigging out.

"For people who are active, it takes a greater crisis to trigger the cortisol response as compared with sedentary people," says Monika R. Fleshner, PhD, a professor of integrative physiology at the University of Colorado at Boulder. "So, now, you can go into a stressful environment and be okay. You can endure a lot more before you kick off a stress response."

Hills also make you happier. Longer, sustained efforts trigger the release of mood-lifting chemicals like endorphins and cannabinoids, which, as the name suggests, are in the same family of chemicals that give pot-smokers their high. Research also shows that regular efforts in the lactate threshold range, which incidentally is the zone in which you perform sustained climbs, can help ward off mood disorders, like depression.

With all that to be gained, it's little wonder that millions of cyclists have made BFFs with mountain passes and the sweet, painful benefits they bring.

THE PATIENCE AND PERSISTENCE PAY OFF

Regardless of where you start your quest, you're embarking on a journey that will be sometimes hard and humbling, occasionally frustrating, and one that requires and rewards patience and persistence. You'll also likely be surprised by what you find along the way.

Case in point: Three riders who made it their personal missions to master climbs for very different reasons. Each took the same approach: Ride up the same gut-busting climb again and again (and again) until they got better. Here's what they found.

Caitlin Giddings had just one wish—to master Stonesthrow, a steep, straight mile-long double-climb (you're not done when you think you are) in the Lehigh Valley region of Pennsylvania that saw her getting spat off the back of her regular group ride. So, she decided to face down this mother every day for 2 weeks straight. "I didn't know what I would find," she says. "Could I actually get faster at it in that amount of time? Would it start to feel easier, or would it become a spirit-crushing slog?"

Her biggest concern was getting bored. That ended up not being a problem. "When I started this challenge, I assumed it would feel monotonous. Instead, the miles felt vastly different, depending on my mood each day. I laughed, I cursed, I lamented layering choices, I felt overcome with the beauty of fall—and on one particularly rough day, I got some bad family news and sobbed in that full-body way that makes you sound like a dying animal. But, I just kept rolling and channeling my pain into digging deeper when the road pointed up. It worked. The only feeling I didn't experience on that godforsaken hill was regret that I was out on my bike."

She also got faster . . . but not at first. "When it came to speed, initially my efforts were pretty discouraging. I felt fast and confident on my first morning up the hill—and then watched myself progressively take on more of the qualities of molasses with each day that passed. But, somewhere around Day 6, I hit a turning point and began to speed up, even on segments that I wasn't trying to work on. It wasn't long before I was pacing myself better up the climb. On my 14th-and-final ascent I captured the second-place QOM [queen of the mountain award] on my nemesis climb. I was also riding more comfortably in pacelines and with my lunch ride group."

Then, there's Todd Scheske, amateur racer and USA Cycling Level 1 Elite Coach with Peaks Coaching Group. As a track racer, his specialty was predominantly sprinting. But, on the road, he had to be able to make it to the end with the front of the pack if he had any prayer of sprinting for a win.

"I was road racing in Venezuela and on the East Coast, going up monsters like Wachusett Mountain [which covers 3.7 miles and climbs 1,162 feet] in Massachusetts, and I'd just get that sinking nervous feeling, knowing that I was going to be in trouble. You know that the climbers are just going to dig into you. If I wanted to race these races, I had to face down these mountains and find a way to succeed at this seemingly insurmountable challenge."

So, one season, Todd did just that. He modified his season to include hill repeat work at least once or twice a week during early season base training. He picked a 4-minute section of one of his hardest local climbs and throttled it over and over to utter and complete failure.

"I would start at this mailbox and charge to the railroad tracks. Then, I would roll back down and allow myself to fully recover—about two to three times as long as the interval itself—and I'd repeat it until I couldn't get within 10 percent of that first effort. That first one was always pretty good, because I'd be full of glycogen and all ambitious. But, they'd just get harder and harder. The first few times out, I could only manage three before I had to pack it in. A few weeks later, it was six. It could turn into an hour to an hour-and-a-half of this. I'd be seeing Jesus on the side of the road halfway through. There were times I would start a seventh effort, and less than halfway through, I couldn't get the pedals around anymore."

It worked—physically and mentally. "I went from being in the small ring and pulling the parachute as soon as a race hit a big climb to being up in the front of the field. I also learned to be more strategic, because I knew I had all these efforts in me. I would break down the climbs into manageable chunks—just make it to that next road sign or driveway; use a bit of sprinting power to throw down just enough acceleration to not get dropped when they started pulling away; and before you know it, you're just a minute from the top, and you can do anything for a minute."

It all paid off with an elite state championship win and fourth at a Masters Nationals Road race in Park City, Utah, where there are lots of long climbs. Like T. J., Todd never learned to love the mountains, per se. But, the lessons have been lasting. "It was an affirmation that hard work works. You can learn to push yourself in places where you're not naturally strong, and break down things that are seemingly insurmountable."

Finally, there's Hunter Allen, founder of the Peaks Coaching Group, headquartered in Bedford, Virginia, who as a decent 185-pound Category 4 (beginner racer) sprinter and criterium rider. Hunter got a rude awakening when he tried his first race with big climbs. "I went out to spend spring break with my uncle in Santa Cruz, California, and raced the Berkeley Hills Road Race. I got spanked so hard. I was like, "Wow, I kind of suck at this!" I came back home and realized that, if I wanted to be good at climbing—and I did—I needed to change my mindset and practice, practice, practice."

And, practice he did. Like Caitlin, Hunter hatched his own personal 2-week training challenge. He would tackle the biggest climb outside of town—The Peaks of Otter (which would later inspire the name of his coaching company and TrainingPeaks training software he co-created)—every day for 2 weeks straight. "No matter how tired, slow, or sore I was, I would do that 30-minute climb every day. and even if I didn't like it, I would convince myself that it was fun!" he says. "I would chant: 'I love climbing. I'm a good climber.' over and over up that damn thing. It was my mantra."

He did get stronger and fitter. But, more importantly, the mental piece really worked. "It was a big paradigm shift for me. I realized that hills made cycling more interesting and fun. It was a great challenge every time. So, I started to seek out other big climbs I could do. I really enjoyed the accomplishment of climbing mountains."

Over the course of 2 years, he got stronger and began joining some of the best climbers in his area on their rides. "I kept pushing myself to train and stay with them longer and longer." He moved up the racing ranks and tweaked his diet, steadily dropping nearly 30 pounds. And then one day, he did it. "I finally beat one of those skinny 130-pound climber dudes! I was like, 'Holy crap, I beat that guy up a mountain!'"

Able to make his mark on the climbs, Hunter enjoyed a few years as a domestic pro rider. Today, he's retired the pro license but not the love of the challenge. "I still have a love of climbing. I still really enjoy getting up the mountain and feeling the accomplishment. It's meaningful."

That meaning is something he hears from clients all the time. "I have a client who's going through a really, really tough time with his business. So, you know I'm telling him it's okay if he doesn't ride every day. But, he says to me, 'You don't realize that cycling is my life right now. It's the only thing I know I can accomplish every day. I can go out and climb that mountain. And, it doesn't matter if I'm putting out 300 watts or just 200 watts; I will get to the top, and I will have accomplished something.'"

THE VIEW FROM ABOVE

It's that sense of accomplishment, the letting go of everything else, and being in the moment of making it up the mountain that makes climbing uniquely transformative. As Sir Edmund Hillary, the first man to stand atop Everest once said, "It's not the mountain we conquer, but ourselves."

That's something Anne Racioppi seeks every time she climbs. So much so that she waxes poetic when asked about her relationship with hill climbing: "It's a time of reflecting, deciphering, understanding, and emptying. Gasping for air in my smallest gear and unable to push the pedals any faster, I can only focus on the loud rhythm of inhale-spinning-exhale-spinning-inhale-spinning-exhale-spinning over and over. Your legs burn from the cadence and effort of the climb. You're tense and loose all at the same time. You're souplesse."

She continues by saying, "When you are pushing your body so hard that you are incapable of hearing sounds or seeing that cute little farmhouse with the rooster mailbox, and you're wholly fixated on breathing and pedaling that *the* moment happens. You separate mind from body. You are free."

When this happens, she says that it's like an "out-of-body experience where you can feel your psyche slowly distancing itself from the chugging machine of your body, and your mind enters a calm and meditative state."

Scientifically speaking, it's also where better health and happiness happen. You already know that the physical act of climbing makes you more physically fit and improves your feeling of well-being. Research also shows that all the fresh air, sunshine, solitude, and sweeping vistas that you soak in as you make your way up and over hills and mountains provide their own unique benefits.

For one, natural light is a known mood-lifter. Just 15 minutes of sunlight a day not only helps you make the vitamin D you need for strong muscles and bones but also it reduces anxiety and depression. As you climb away from the hectic, often-cluttered urban and suburban landscapes where many of us live and work, your mind gets a reprieve from the constant, nearly numbing stimulation that can cause what scientists call cognitive fatigue. You clear your mind as you climb, which is why some of your best ideas—like Einstein's theory of relativity—often come while you're on your bike.

Other research has found that spending more time in scenic environments, especially open blue skies and mountainous landscapes is linked to better health, regardless of other key factors like employment and socioeconomic status. Just 15 to 20 minutes outdoors has been found to boost mood and energy levels. Heck, simply daydreaming about yourself out there climbing through oaks and pines is good for your health, according to a study that found levels of your feel-good brain hormone serotonin rise even when you're just imagining yourself outdoors or recalling some previous outing.

Combine all these benefits of being in the great outdoors with those that come from the physical exertion of getting there by bike and climbing lots of hills is like hitting a mental and physical health jackpot—well worth all the effort.

2 | PHYSICS

Cycling success lies in the forces of the universe.

▶ **THE HARDEST PART OF** most tasks is just getting started. And, if you're sitting at the Marin Circle fountain at the bottom of Marin Avenue in Berkeley, California—a ¾-mile stretch of pavement that averages 16 percent and tops out at 25 percent before you can catch your breath over the crest on Grizzly Peak Boulevard—you know all too well how true that is, when you're behind your bars peering up an incredibly steep incline.

It's hard because you have to overcome some formidable forces of the universe, including rolling resistance (actually not such a biggie), air friction (kind of a big deal), and gravity (a whopper, when it comes to climbing). What does it take to overcome all this? I'm not a physicist. So I asked one: Joel Fajans, PhD, who is a professor of physics at University of California Berkeley and also an avid cyclist.

Rolling resistance, which includes the friction of your tires against the ground as well as chain friction on your gears, is the first force you encounter

> ## 🏁 FUN FACT
>
> At low speeds, before the wind starts kicking you in the face, bicycles are super efficient. It's been said that a person on a bike is the most efficient transport system (for weight over distance). Better than any vehicle, bird, or fish.

and have to overcome, but it's so easy that pretty much anyone can do it. You need only to generate a few watts, and you're in motion. The faster you go, the more important air resistance becomes. "Shortly above 10 mph, air resistance quickly dominates, but the total power you need at that point is still pretty low—about 40 watts," says Dr. Fajans.

Air resistance gets harder with increasing speed. "To go from 15 mph to 16 mph requires the power to increase from about 100 to 117 watts, a 17-percent increase," explains Dr. Fajans. If you've ever found yourself huffing and puffing too hard to swear at a riding buddy who is *just* a bit faster (and won't slow the hell down), this is why. "If their natural speed is only 1 mph faster than yours, you have to increase your power by 17 percent. Consider that heart rate is roughly proportional to power. So, that's like going from 120 beats per minute to 140 beats per minute. Not easy." At race pace speeds? That's where the phrase "aero is everything" was born. "At 20 mph, a 1-mph increase requires the power to go from 208 to 237 watts, a 14-percent increase, or say a heart beat increase from 150 to 170 beats per minute. *Really* not easy." At that point, rolling resistance is nearly irrelevant.

Now, let's add some incline, which is a matter of figuring your "rise to run," or how many vertical feet you travel for every 100 feet you go forward. If you go back to your high-school geometry, it's like pedaling up the hypotenuse of a right triangle where the x axis is a flat plane on the Earth, and the y axis is a giant fireman's pole to the sky). Just tack a percentage sign on that vertical distance, and that's the grade: If you climb 7 feet as you go forward 100 feet, that's a 7-percent gradient.

WATTS UP?

In physics speak, the power required to climb a hill increases linearly in proportion to the hill's grade, the rider's velocity, and the rider's (and their bike's) weight, explains our good professor. Simply put, the steeper the mother, the harder it is to go fast, especially if you're not whippet-thin.

Let's say you're a 150-pound rider with a 20-pound bike, and you want to see if you can nab the King or Queen of the Mountain spot on Strava (a popular training app that lets you compare your ride performances to other users and awards you crowns for fastest times) up the hotly contested $\frac{1}{4}$-mile, 5-percent ramp up to the local retirement home on the hill. You need to be prepared to produce some serious wattage, because you're going to have to do a lot of work for every additional fraction of mph.

Let's say the fastest time and speed on the leaderboard is just less than 1 minute and just over 19 mph. An effort of that magnitude will take 530 watts to achieve. To put it into perspective for those who don't train with power, four-time Tour de France winner Chris Froome cranks out about 520 watts when he launches attacks on his rivals in the mountains. So, you'd need to churn out a little more than that (enough to power your hedge trimmer). Not an easy feat.

Now, let's tilt this sucker upward to 18 percent. Hitting double digits in miles per hour for any length of time is pretty much out of the question, as you'd need to crank out well over 600 watts. Again, for perspective, the average trained cyclist hits 600 watts in a full-bore sprint; they may manage a third that much up a sustained climb. Going just half that—5 mph—demands a steady 300 watts, considerably more than most recreational cyclists can sustain for more than a few minutes.

Which is precisely why sometimes it's easier to jog (if you have no bike) or give up the ghost and get off and push your bike when the hill is relentlessly, stupidly steep, explains Dr. Fajans. "For that 150-pound person, saving the 20 pounds of bicycle increases their speed by about 13 percent," he says. "For the 150-pound person *on* the bicycle, the problem becomes balance. Bicycles are easier to ride at speed. Near to, and certainly below 5 mph, they are rather

➚ HOW LONG IT TAKES TO CLIMB MOUNT VENTOUX

One of the most storied climbs in pro cycling—for its stark moonscape summit, where strong, violent winds can add considerable air resistance to an already taxing nearly 9-percent average grade—is Mount Ventoux, which overlooks the Rhone Valley in France. It's been included in the Tour de France more than 15 times since 1951.

Professional cyclists can average over 400 watts on this monstrous 13.5-mile mountain. Average cyclists will put out less than half that wattage—closer to 195 watts. That means the fastest guys in the flock (who hit the summit in an average of 58:30 minutes) can climb Ventoux almost twice by the time you reach the top.

---

hard to ride. So at slow speeds, one is fighting for balance, which wastes a good bit of energy that you don't have in that moment in time."

So, just how steep is too freakin' steep to make it up with two wheels? This one intrigued Dr. Fajans, who had never considered the question. "The ultimate limit comes from the requirement that the center of mass of the person and bike has to be in front of the contact point of the rear wheel on the ground," he says. In plain English, if your center of gravity is around your belly button, you need to move more and more forward on the bike to keep your center of gravity over the rear wheel as the climb gets steeper. That's why, when you look at pictures from ginormous hill climbs like Mount Washington in New Hampshire (which averages 12 percent and tops out at 22 percent in the final corkscrew to the summit, where snapped chains and toppled riders aren't uncommon), they're hunkered *way* over the front of their handlebars to maintain that sweet spot for weight over the rear wheel.

"I'd guess that the center of mass is up about 115 centimeters [45 inches] from the ground, and one can lean forward enough to push the center of mass forward of the rear wheel contact by 65 centimeters [25 inches]. This gives a maximum climbing angle of about 30 degrees," calculates Dr. Fajans. For the Southern Californians in the crowd, LA's steepest streets (and there are some doozies) top out at 33 percent, which has caused trucks to lose their cargo; the US Postal Service leaves all residents' mail in one big bin at the bottom of the hill.

Where all this gets really problematic is in the sheer amount of power it takes to keep the pedals turning on that great of a grade. "The power required to maintain 5 mph is 500 watts," says Dr. Fajans. "That isn't doable for most people. At a more realistic 250 watts, the speed is 2.5 mph. It is really difficult to ride this slowly. And, that's if you were riding at a constant speed. During the power phase of your pedal stroke (when the pedals are

⊘ COASTING UPHILL AND SWEATING GOING DOWNHILL?

"Not another climb… wait? … Why am I going so fast and barely working?" Those were my exact thoughts on one stretch of road during a ride through the middle of Montana many moons ago. It was my first multiday charity ride. I was pretty torched and ready to be done, and I couldn't tell if I was hallucinating or in some upside-down world where the universe's gravitational forces were flipped. Turns out, like the slanted floors in a fun house, it was an optical illusion.

Psychologists explain that these illusions are produced inside our brains when the surrounding landscape—trees, walls, and so forth—is tilted in such a way that it appears we're going uphill when we're actually going downhill, and vice versa. This phenomenon can be powerful. An example is Magnetic Hill in Moncton, New Brunswick, which the Canadian province's website hails as an "amazing natural phenomenon" where you can "sit back and be amazed as you drive your car to the bottom of Magnetic Hill, take your foot off the brake, and roll back uphill." It has been a tourist attraction for nearly a century and sounds like an awesome place to go by bike.

approximately horizontal) you tend to accelerate. That tends to pull the front wheel off the ground."

CATEGORIZING CLIMBS

Given our little physics lesson, clearly when your riding mates tell you that a climb is "just a half-mile long," they're not really sharing useful information. Because, hey, it's super-short, how bad could it be? Right? Right. . . . Let's look at a little country lane called Goat Hill, for example. It's a soul-crusher on one of our annual charity rides in Pennsylvania that's just 0.5 mile long, but it has an average gradient of 15 percent and hits a nearly vertical 31.4 percent at its steepest pitch. Oh, and it's unpaved, often rutted, and sometimes soft. Many cyclists are simply forced to walk.

Sometimes, you'll see signs—often intended for truckers, but quite useful for cyclists—that will tell you the grade of an upcoming climb, particularly if it is prolonged or well-traveled. If there's no signage, your cycling computer likely has a feature that allows you to see the gradient in real time (or pretty close to it). In the absence of either of these things, you can generally get a sense of what gradient you're on, once you know how various inclines feel beneath your wheels. I've seen various descriptions of hill inclines over the years, and here's my take.

- **0 percent:** Dead flat. Easy peasy. Unless you're battling a headwind, this is smooth sailing.
- **1 to 2 percent:** This is what you'd call "false flat," because it looks pretty flat... but it's not. These can be mentally draining when they go on for long stretches of straight road, because you're not really climbing, so there's no "top" as a reward.
- **3 to 4 percent:** Slight climb. The effort is similar to riding into a headwind. Totally manageable, but grinding away up these grades can be fatiguing— and downright annoying—if they refuse to let up or even undulate a little.
- **5 to 6 percent:** There's no doubt that you're climbing, as your speed slows by

about half. But it's manageable. Heck, even playful. These are the types of climbs you can "dance on the pedals" with, alternating between sitting and standing.
- **7 to 8 percent:** These are decidedly less playful. Here, you'll find yourself bowing over your bars as if in a spell of prayer to find a few fresh muscle fibers to make it to the top.
- **9 to 10 percent:** Yeah, you're not just bent over your bars, you're actually pulling out a few Hail Marys each time you round a bend convinced it's going to let up, but it doesn't.
- **11 to 12 percent:** Now you're praying. Just. One. More. Gear. You chew on your bar tape and maybe start to tack ever so slightly.
- **13 to 15 percent:** Soul-searching territory. Your mind worries over the big whys? "Why did I take up this sport? Why do I think this is fun? Why do they make roads like this?"
- **16 to 18 percent:** Hey, look, it's Jesus on the side of the road waving to you! You'd wave back, but you'd topple over if you dared to take a hand off the hoods.
- **18 percent and above:** Speaking of Jesus . . . any climb that kicks into this territory will definitely present some come-to-Jesus (or deity of choice) moments—and you'll feel like you've absolutely reached the pearly gates or Nirvana when it's over.

But gradient isn't the only variable that influences how hard a hill will be to climb. Other factors that come into play:

AVERAGE GRADE: As the name implies, the average grade of a climb is the percentage that it goes up over the distance of the climb. But, very few real-world climbs are straight up-and-down affairs. So, a climb that is consistently 7 percent will feel very different from one that has equal portions at 2 percent and 14 percent (an extreme example, but you get the point). Which is harder? That depends on the rest of the factors.

STEEPEST GRADE: Back to the 31.4 percent Goat Hill mentioned earlier. That section alone, especially since it comes in the midst of a climb that is nearly consistently in the double digits gradient-wise, makes this an enormously difficult climb. The same could be said for a 7-mile climb that meanders at a leg-fatiguing 5 to 6 percent before finishing you off at 10 to 12 percent.

DISTANCE: Anyone who's ever tried to keep their voice from cracking and betraying the swelling panic inside while asking, "How much farther to the top?" knows that distance is a huge factor when ranking a hill's difficulty. The average grade of Mount Lemmon on the northern edge of Tucson is only 4.1 percent, but the ascent is *28.5 miles long*. That's very important information.

INCREASE IN ALTITUDE FROM BOTTOM TO TOP: How many feet of elevation you gain from the time the climb starts to its summit. This one can be deceptive, though. There's a massive difference between climbing Waterrock Knob in North Carolina and Route 475 in New Mexico, even if both gain roughly 3,500 feet of elevation and average 4- to 5-percent grade over 13 to 15 miles. Waterrock tops out at about 6,300 feet above sea level—which is roughly where the 475 starts before you soar into the clouds above 10,000 feet. Altitude makes all the difference.

THE TOTAL ALTITUDE AT THE TOP: The thin air at high altitude seriously saps your power and makes your legs beg for mercy on even relatively gentle climbs. Again, thank (or blame) physics. As you climb higher, the air pressure becomes lower, so oxygen molecules spread out, leaving you with less O_2 in every breath you take. That makes your heart work harder, so a climb you might have pedaled up at 150 beats per minute will now force your pump to crank into the 160s.

ROAD CONDITIONS: A sweet, smooth, newly paved road—unless slick with rain—will take less energy to climb than a stretch of chopped up tarmac that keeps bucking you off your line. Deep gravel or pea pebbles over hard pack will be even worse.

If you're ranking climbs along a specific route, you also can factor in just how tired you're going to be when you hit a certain incline. For instance, there's a little kicker off Main Street that I need to take back to my house after rides. It's not even a $\frac{1}{4}$ mile long, but it tops out at 9.7 percent, and sometimes it feels like the hardest push of the day, just because I'm fully spent by the time I need to get over that hump.

Though it's far from an exact science, all those factors get tossed into the matrix to rate climbs according to the following categories of difficulty from easiest to most arduous. There are no hard-and-fast rules, but, according to the pro cycling website *Cycling Today*, this is how the Tour de France defines their climbs:

Category 4: These are relatively short and not too steep. This would include a climb that's about a mile to a mile-and-a-quarter long at a 5-percent grade or one that is twice that long at a 2- to 3-percent grade.

Category 3: These are a little steeper or a little longer. For instance, it could be a mile-long climb that includes pitches at 10 percent or a 5- to 6-mile climb that grinds away at 4 to 5 percent.

Category 2: Here's where stuff gets pretty hard. You're looking at a 9- to 10-mile climb at about 4 percent or a climb that's a third of the distance but twice as steep.

Category 1: Formerly known as the highest category of climb, Cat 1s include anything from 5 miles at a leg-buckling 8 percent to a dozen miles of soul-sucking 5 percent.

Hors Catégorie: French for stupid hard, or "above category," these behemoths are a quad-searing mix of long and steep, which could be a 6-mile climb with an average grade of 7 to 8 percent or a 15-mile monster that turns the screws at 6 percent or steeper.

Finally, when you're eyeballing just how tough a route will be, you want to add up the total vertical distance you'll be climbing over the entire ride. This number can take you by surprise sometimes, especially in places that you wouldn't define as mountainous. In fact, as we'll discuss in Chapter 10, relentlessly hilly places where you rack up 1,000 or so vertical feet for every 10 miles that come at you 50 to 150 punchy feet at a time can wear you down quicker than meandering your way up a few monstrous California climbs that never stretch above 6 percent and that allow you to settle into a rhythm to spin your way up and over with ample recovery on the other side.

One final word on physics comes from T. J. Klausutis, the big man on a bike we met in the last chapter. "My best advice is to understand physics. She can be a harsh mistress, but you have to understand how to dance with her. Big people will have a huge advantage downhill and in the flats because they are working with gravity and can generate so much power. Learn how to put power down judiciously over long periods of time according to your body type," which leads us into the next chapter.

3 | GOATS AND GRINDERS

You can maximize your uphill skills, no matter your size.

▶ **THE BIGGER THE MOUNTAINS,** the smaller their conquerors tend to be. As explored in the previous chapter, that's just the laws of physics, or more specifically a concept known as power-to-weight—how many watts you can produce divided by how much you weigh. This ratio isn't very important on flat land, but on a climb, especially a relatively steep one, it's a major factor. That's because lighter riders can overcome Earth's gravitational pull and scamper their way up the incline with relatively lower power output (though a higher absolute power-to-weight ratio) compared to heavier cyclists.

So, no. You can't defy physics. Yet that doesn't mean that you should throw your hands up and declare that you'll never be a climber simply because your jersey tag says L . . . or has an X (or more than one X) in front of that letter. True, larger riders may never win a King or Queen of the Mountain polka-dotted jersey in a professional Grand Tour (an honor that is bestowed on roughly 0.0000001 percent of the population—my rough estimate anyway), but that doesn't mean that they can't be good climbers, or, even more importantly, really enjoy—even relish—climbing.

Also, let's not forget that every equation has two sides. In this case, the focus on weight narrowly views climbing from one side of the equation—that which favors the natural mountain goats. It overlooks the fact that many a cyclist has left their mark in the mountains simply by being more powerful and grinding it out. With the right techniques, body position, and strategy, you can make the most of every watt, no matter what you weigh.

IT'S NOT JUST THE SIZE OF THE RIDER BUT THE POWER IN THE PEDAL STROKE

For the sake of scientific discussion—and because the stats are pretty cool to know—let's first look at how power-to-weight plays out in terms of cycling success in the mountains. In an interview with coaching guru Joe Friel, creator of *The Cyclist's Training Bible* series, Friel calculated that the fastest male recreational riders—you know the ones you find hogging up the top of the Strava leaderboards where you live—generally carry in the range of 2.1 to 2.4 pounds per inch, topping out at about 168 pounds for a 5′10″ guy. The speediest female amateurs carry 1.9 to 2.2 pounds per inch, which tops out at 143 pounds for a 5′5″ woman.

In the elite ranks, climbing specialists are considerably lighter. Top elite male climbers (we're talking Tour pros here) generally carry less than 2 pounds of body weight per inch of height, and elite women carry about 1.8 or fewer pounds per inch. That means that same 5′10″ man would need to slim down to 140 pounds, and that 5′5″ female would need to tip the scales at 117 pounds. Real-world references bear that out. Alberto Contador a world-renowned Spanish summit bagger, carries 137 pounds on his 5′9″ frame. Marti Shea, who holds the course record and won a staggering 11 titles up the infamous Mount Washington Auto Road Bicycle Hillclimb in New Hampshire reports that 110 pounds on her 5′4″ frame was her best fighting weight.

Still, all of this needs perspective. For one, those figures are honing in on an extremely narrow population, and even within that extremely small group of high-ranking pros, you have a fair share of riders on the heavier side of the spectrum who can generate enough power to overcome a few extra pounds. And, let's face it, most of us are also pretty happy with less than record-breaking performances. Case in point (and fun fact), when I Googled Marti Shea to check her stats, I was greeted by a picture of myself next to her on the 2010 Mount Washington podium. I'd won my age group and gotten third place overall that year, and I was completely and utterly over the moon. Could I ever break the record? Not in this lifetime, and not at 130 nonpetite pounds. I would have to cut off part of an appendage to hit her weight. But, I still consider that race a resounding success, and one of my proudest cycling accomplishments.

Let's also talk actual time penalty for excess pounds. Every 5 pounds of body weight you carry over your ideal weight will slow you down about 15 to 20 seconds per mile up a 4- to 5-percent climb. So, you'll be about 45 seconds to a minute slower up a 5-kilometer climb than a rider who's at their power-to-weight sweet spot—not so bad. It starts to add up, though, as the climbing feet mount, of course. Out West, where you'll find some 15-mile monsters, those at ideal power-to-weight will have 3 to 4 minutes to pull out their phones and Instagram the moment before their friends with less-than-ideal power-to-weight ratios reach the summit.

The key words here, however, are "ideal" and "sweet spot." Fact is, we're all built differently. If you have a small skeletal frame, you're going to be naturally lighter than someone built more broadly. It can be unrealistic, if not downright counterproductive, to try to drop down to an unnaturally light weight, especially if you have a medium or large skeletal frame and/or tend toward the muscular side.

For reference, most of us can slot our overall build into one of three general categories (recognizing that there are a wide variety of shapes and sizes even within these categories).

- **ECTOMORPH:** You tend to be long-limbed and not particularly muscular.
- **MESOMORPH:** You are muscular and tend to be proportionally built.
- **ENDOMORPH:** You are generally more heavyset.

PUT YOUR POWER TO THE TEST

Pounds-to-inches is a pretty good ballpark for power-to-weight estimates. If you have a power meter, however, you can calculate it the way that exercise physiologists and other coaching pros do—by measuring the maximum power you can sustain for an extended period of time.

The standard test used in the lab or the field is to perform a 20-minute time trial (after a thorough warm up of at least 20 minutes)—keeping your effort as high as you can sustain—on a slight uphill grade or false flat. No hill at your disposal? Simulate the test on a flat road or trainer, using enough resistance so you feel like you're on a gentle uphill grade. Avoid rolling roads, because the downhill sections will lower your overall power number. Record the average wattage you produce, then divide the watts by your morning body weight in kilograms (pounds divided by 2.2). So, if you weigh 180 pounds (82 kilograms) and you average 270 watts, your power-to-weight ratio is 3.3 watts per kilogram.

To score a top spot on a professional squad, that number would need to be above 6 watts per kilogram, and you'd have to sustain that output for more than 20 to 30 minutes. If you're going to conquer an Alpine climb, you're talking an hour. Beginner cyclists usually pull in the range of 2.5 to 3.2 watts per kilogram for men, and 2.1 to 2.8 for women. Fast recreational riders produce wattage in the range of 3.7 to 4.4 for men, and 3.2 to 3.8 for women. To be competitive in 30- to 60-minute time trials and hill climbs, men need to push it above the 4.5 range, and women should come in closer to 4.

If you're cranking out 2.9 and want to hit 3.9, look at your weight first. If you're carrying a bit of a spare tire around your torso, it's probably easiest to pick up some speed, especially up those climbs, by shedding a few pounds. If your weight is in a good place, work on your power. Most cyclists benefit from a combination of the two. (See Chapters 5 and 8 for action plans.)

How much can you expect to improve? Through high-intensity training, you can raise your wattage by 5 to 7 percent over the course of a season. One surefire strategy: Climb for 10 to 30 minutes at or near lactate threshold heart rate (about an 8 on a 1-to-10 rated perceived exertion scale (RPE), with 10 being all-out) twice a week. If you want to improve your ratio, work at lowering the weight part of the equation.

Muscle tissue is dense, so someone who is muscular is always going to be heavier than someone who is less so. But, as you might have guessed, that person may also produce more horsepower. This is where performance can't be confined to a number on a scale. You need strength to push the gear, leg speed to turn it over, and a strong, finely tuned cardiovascular engine to sustain that effort. Your sweet spot is a body weight that optimizes all that.

What does that mean in terms of your body type? If you're an ectomorph, you might have a low scale number but still not maximum strength. We coaches and trainers have all worked with light riders who get smoked up climbs or are not climbing to their potential because they have low power. When they hit the gym for some squats and leg presses (see Chapter 5 for more on this), they develop that strength. It may inch the scale a bit higher but with positive, not negative, results.

"I've seen people get too light and lose power, even among the more natural climbers I work with," says Todd Scheske of Peaks Coaching Group, who you may remember from Chapter 1, transformed his own heavy-sprinter self into a power climber. That includes Victoria Di Savino, 38, of Buffalo, who won Mount Washington in 2016 with a time of 1:07:32, after a second-place finish the year before. "We had her get into the gym and put on a couple pounds of muscle for Mount Washington, and she was *flying*. Remember what you're chasing. You're chasing speed. Nobody cares about your watts and kilograms during competition. You just care who is powerful and efficient," says Scheske.

"Light people can climb, but you have to be powerful, too," says Di Savino. "For one, if your upper body is weak, your climbing suffers. Also, people don't consider the relative weight of their bikes. My bike is much heavier in comparison to my weight than the same bike would be for a larger rider. I need to be stronger to carry that weight up the hill. You should concentrate on being strong, not skinny."

Now, if you're an endomorph? The rules may change a bit. Your muscle is your engine, but you don't need chest and arm muscles like an NFL fullback to turn cranks. In that case, too much muscle literally weighs you down. While you shouldn't seek to deliberately lose muscle, you may want to avoid gaining it where you don't need it, like your upper body. To a lesser extent, the same can be true for mesomorphs who also can have the propensity to gain muscle mass easily.

SITTING OR STANDING: FINDING YOUR BEST FORM ON THE PEDALS

No matter your current weight, technique is a hugely important—and an often-overlooked—way to conserve energy, while producing the watts you need for the job at hand, like, say, working your way up a 5-mile, mixed-gradient, leg-burner of a climb. It's also immediately beneficial. So, while you'll find training and nutrition advice for making long-term jumps in climbing speed, improving your form will deliver instant gratification.

Technique-related queries are also among the most commonly asked questions that come across my desk. For instance, take Glenn Turner, a powerful all-arounder—his riding interests include cyclocross and mountain bike racing—who describes himself as "not having the typical climber's physique." Glenn loves climbs. He just wants to hone his technique to be better. He has the mental peace (more on that in Chapter 6), but tactics still leave him puzzled. "I love all climbs," he says. "It's all about pushing yourself to the point of collapse, and then digging deeper and saying, 'I have this.' But, I'm always asking myself, 'Should I spin or should I power my way to the top? How can I use my strengths best?'" Great questions. Here are the answers.

WHEN AND HOW TO CLIMB SEATED

Generally speaking, you should climb seated most of the time, standing only to stretch out your legs and release tension in your back or to attack a steep pitch, summit, or rival. Seated climbing saves energy, especially if you're a larger rider. With your rear planted on your saddle, your body weight is fully supported on the bike and your leg muscles can expend all their energy pushing the pedals and powering you up the grade. Here's how to make the most of every stroke.

TORSO: Relax! No seriously. RELAX! The mountain is like a tiger. You don't want to show it you're afraid or it'll pounce all over you. It also saps vital energy as you white-knuckle the bars and raise your shoulders up to your ears. So, place your hands loosely on the top of the bars or the hoods, relax your shoulders, open your chest, and engage your core muscles to provide a solid pedaling platform. As the climb gets steeper, pull back a bit on the bars to send more power through your torso and into your pedals.

ARMS: Keep your arms loosely bent and close to your sides, with elbows slightly flared (but not jutting out like chicken wings) just past your knuckles. Even on a mountain bike or flat-bar bike, you'll want to keep your elbows tucked in a bit to keep your core tight and produce more power pulling through the bars. Grasp the bar firmly but gently.

BUTT: Move it around, especially on long climbs, as different positions engage different muscles. Shift back toward the rear of the saddle to employ more glute muscles—this is especially useful when the going gets steep, and you've run out of gears, so you need to put that much more power into every pedal stroke. Scoot forward toward the nose to engage more quads. Slide back to center to use a bit of everything. By shifting your weight—and the workload—around, you'll keep your legs fresher overall.

FEET: Many riders fritter away valuable watts at this key junction by pedaling up a climb with their toes pointed down. Your feet are the platform that puts power into your pedals. You want that platform to be as powerful as possible. That means keeping your feet flat and driving downward through your heels or the midfoot with your ankles locked to help transfer that power. Keeping your heels low also engages more hamstring and glute muscles and puts less stress on your calves. (This is an easier, more-natural foot position to achieve at lower cadences like when you're climbing. As your cadence rises on the flats, it's natural for your heel to be slightly higher.)

WHEN AND HOW TO CLIMB OUT OF THE SADDLE

Sometimes, you just have to get out of the saddle. Standing allows you to push back against gravity with all your weight, so you get a short surge of power (smaller riders typically stand more for this reason—they need the extra assist). That said, when you stand, you force your legs to carry more of your body weight, so they have to work harder, which ultimately uses about 10 percent more energy and sends your heart rate 5 to 10 percent higher (also why larger riders tend to stand less—it's that much more work).

TORSO: Keep your back straight and hips back over the bottom bracket as you stand. Often, riders will pitch their bodies too far forward toward their front wheels, which causes the back tire to break traction and skid. For steep, double-digit grades, you'll need to hinge forward and lower your upper body over your bars to keep your weight centered (and the front wheel in contact with the ground), but your hips should remain back over the bottom bracket.

ARMS: While you want your torso to remain stable and steady up a steep climb, you'll often need to gently rock the bike beneath you to put down additional power up a steep grade, such as when the climb kicks through a hairpin or you see the top and you're ready to get this thing over with! Place your hands on the hoods (or outer parts of the bars on a flat-bar bike), and rhythmically torque the bike beneath you to accelerate it through a steep pitch. It will feel as though you're gently pushing the bike side to side in time with your pedal stroke, so as your right leg extends, you're pressing into the left side of the bars and vice versa.

BUTT: Your hips should be over the saddle with your weight over the bottom bracket, so the nose of your saddle brushes the back of your thighs. Depending on the pitch of the climb and your body type, you may decide to stand tall out of the saddle, allowing your full body weight to come down on the pedals. Or, you can hover, keeping your upper body relatively parallel to the bike but lifting your butt off the saddle for just a little extra oomph.

FEET: As with seated climbing, you want to leverage those powerful platforms by keeping your feet relatively flat as you drive with your mid- to rear foot.

WHAT'S THE BEST PEDALING CADENCE?

Cadence is a story of your legs versus your lungs, because there are only two ways to increase your power and, hence, go faster up that climb. You can put more actual force on the pedal—bigger gear, slower pedaling style—or you can increase the number of times you turn the pedals per minute—lower gear, high-speed spinning style. The former puts more stress on your leg muscles but doesn't tax your aerobic system very much, so your heart rate stays relatively low. The latter is a very aerobic effort, so your cardiovascular system needs to kick into high gear, which drives up your heart rate and makes you huff and puff.

Despite what you may have heard, there is no magical number that is just right for every rider, and the cadence you choose depends on your fitness level, muscle fiber type, general build, and so forth. In general, bigger, more-muscular riders can get away with a harder gear and lower cadence; however, no matter your size, erring toward a brisker cadence, when possible, will help you be more successful for a few reasons.

For one, your heart and lungs will outlast your legs. Sinking into a low cadence, which is anything below 70 rpm, is akin to leg pressing your way up the mountain. How many leg presses can you do before your quads catch fire? Exactly. And, once your legs start burning, you're going to have to slow down significantly to try to let them recover, which is tough when you're still on a climb.

Hard-gear, low-cadence climbing also doesn't allow much wiggle room for changes in pitch or speed. So, if the hill suddenly gets steeper, you're forced to try to make a shift under load (how chains meet their snapping demise). Likewise, if the group you're riding with starts to pick up the pace, you're pretty much screwed because you're already applying near max effort and accelerating is out of the question.

Climbing in a slightly easier gear and quicker cadence gives you more flexibility to meet the demands of the climb. You can accelerate a little bit when you need to go just a bit faster or you can shift down and push a bigger gear, if you need to bring your heart rate down. Mashing monster gears also places more torque on your knees. Try to stay above 70 rpm, aiming for a range of 75 to 90 rpm.

Like your body position on the bike, don't be afraid to intentionally mix up your cadence on a sustained climb. By alternating between faster and slower cadences, you give your body (and mind) a break from cranking along like a metronome.

⬈ ANTICIPATE THE SHIFT

Maintaining your cadence requires using your gears early and often. That means being sensitive to all the climbing cues that indicate you're going to want an easier gear. The most obvious one is pressure on your pedals. As soon as you feel the pressure starting to increase, shift in response to keep your cadence constant. This includes shifting into a harder gear anytime the hill relaxes, to keep your effort steady and to keep you from spinning out. You also can shift with your eyes—as you see the ground undulating ahead of you, shifting in rhythm with it will allow you to maximize your momentum without spinning out or slowing down. Whatever you do, always shift before you stand. Click into a harder gear and stand as your power foot (generally the foot on the same side as your dominant hand) comes to the top of the pedal stroke. This will push you forward and boost your momentum (as well as keep the bike from kicking back into some unlucky rider close to your wheel).

HARD SHOULD YOU GO?

This is a biggie and one that can be a work in progress for your entire climbing life (i.e., we all still blow it sometimes). The sweet spot for climbing success is keeping your effort right below your lactate threshold level. Once you go above that threshold, your body is producing lactate faster than your muscles can use it. Your heart beats faster, your breathing becomes labored, and your legs alight with that familiar searing sensation that forces you to come to a crawl and try to recover.

The ideal climbing intensity is just below threshold (where your legs start to burn). To find it, ride a hill as hard as your legs will allow (you should be able to sustain it for more than 30 seconds), then back it down about 10 percent. This gives you a reserve to dig into so you can handle changes in pace and pitch without popping. If you're already at threshold, you have nowhere to go but down.

If you train with a heart-rate monitor or power meter, you can keep yourself honest by watching your metrics. You shouldn't be working harder than 85 to 94 percent of your max heart rate, or MHR, and 90 to 105 percent functional threshold power, or FTP (more on those in Chapter 4). That's a 7 to 8 on a scale of 1 to 10. Your breathing is short, fast, and rhythmic but, most importantly, controlled. Once you reach that point where you're huffing and puffing hard, and your breathing feels like it's anything but in your own control, you've crossed over threshold and into the red.

For long climbs, or when you know you're going to be climbing all day, backing the effort down to tempo—or intensive endurance—pace is even better. Here, your breathing is just slightly labored. You're sitting about 75 to 84 percent of MHR and 75 to 90 percent FTP, or about a 5 to 6 on the 10-point effort scale. It's what you'd describe as comfortably hard.

When in doubt, start a climb at a pace that feels easier than it should. You can always pick up the pace as you near the top. If you're climbing with a group, and you're not among the strongest climbers in the group and concerned about losing them before you get to the top, position yourself in the front of the pack at the start of the climb. That way, you'll give yourself a bit of a fallback zone to slow your pace and recover your legs here and there without being dropped too far off the back.

FOUR TYPES OF CLIMBS—
AND HOW TO ATTACK THEM

Climbing is like dancing: You want to move to the rhythm of each unique ascent to maximize your forward momentum (and ultimate enjoyment), just as each piece of music is unique and inspires different moves. Here are a few techniques for "dancing" up each hill and mountainside, regardless of the length and grade.

ROCK THE ROLLERS. Rollers are sometimes referred to as sprinter's climbs, because they're all about pure power and maintaining momentum. For this reason, bigger riders often like these best—it's the kind of climbing

(continued on page 36)

PLAYING WITH FIRE

"Oh, my God.... How is that guy still right behind me up this hill?!"

Those were my exact thoughts during an organized ride a little while back. It was the third in a series of spring classics that I do each year along the Pennsylvania–New Jersey border. They're notoriously hard and hilly, with elevation profiles that look like an EKG readout (maybe your own while you're out there!) as you hit one incessantly steep, gravel road climb after another... with scant recovery in between. I was 48 miles into an 80-mile, 6,000-plus feet climb when I hit the Narrows, a skinny stretch of goat path that averages 13 percent but kicks up to 30 percent for a few seconds, making you feel you might fall over (one guy did, actually), then really never relents until you reach the top about a half mile later. The man behind me was sucking wind like a runaway train. I've never actually heard anything like it.

He drifted a few bike lengths back, but crested the monster, and rolled up by my side moments later, still huffing and puffing hard. This process repeated itself up and over multiple climbs, and I found myself wondering just how many matches my newfound friend could burn before he would be completely torched. So, I started counting. The answer was nine (and it was really pretty impressive—no way I could've gone that deep over and over and hung on that long). As we hit the final few miles of ascent, before we were rewarded with a blissful few miles of descent, he completely disappeared from view. He was simply all out of matches, which is a concept that is key for hill-climbing success.

When coaches and riders talk about burning matches, they're referring to those efforts that force you to dig really deep. Most of us know when we've burned one, because it hurts! Hunter Allen (from Chapter 1), founder of the Peaks Coaching Group, a co-developer of TrainingPeaks coaching software, and co-author of *Training and Racing with a Power Meter*—so an extremely analytical guy—actually sat down and quantified it a few years back. "You can define it as an effort in which you push past your threshold power by at least 20 percent and hold it there for at least 1 minute," he says. You can extrapolate from there with the understanding that lower intensity (but above threshold) efforts can still burn matches, if you hold them long enough. For instance, if you're chasing someone up a slight grade for 10 minutes, hovering just 10 percent over threshold, you're still gonna burn a match. Allen shared the chart below to illustrate what match-burning looks like at various above-threshold intensities. (You can also get super-techy and use TrainingPeaks software to track your matches.)

You have only so many matches at your disposal on any given day, depending on your fitness and state of recovery, and every rider's matchbook is different. Some have just a little pack, and others seemingly have an industrial-size box. What's important is that you get a sense of your match-burning ability, especially on hilly rides, where recovery can be hard to come by. If you know you'll be going up and over hills all day, you want to keep that matchbook filled, so you can light it up at the end of the ride, instead of going up in flames.

TIME	PERCENTAGE OVER THRESHOLD POWER	POWER NEEDED TO BURN A "MATCH" ASSUMING 300 THRESHOLD POWER
1 minute	20+	360 watts
5 minutes	15-20	360-345 watts
10 minutes	8-12	324-336 watts
20 minutes	0-8	300-324 watts

Courtesy of Hunter Allen, founder of the Peaks Coaching Group, a co-developer of TrainingPeaks coaching software, and co-author of Training and Racing with a Power Meter.

where they can often dust the smaller climbing specialists. To tackle them, crank up the pace as you approach the base of the roller, shift into an easier gear as you hit the grade, and gradually increase your effort as you pedal upward. (You might slide a hair into the red here, which is okay so long as it's just a little, as rollers are generally short, but you'll have a chance to recover on the other side.) Stay seated until your cadence drops, then stand to power over the top, shifting, as necessary, to maintain momentum. If you're working through a series of rollers, resist the urge to coast down the other side. Instead, keep pedaling and build as much easy speed on the downslope as possible to propel you into the next kicker.

SIT AND SPIN ON THE LONG STEADIES. Long, steady climbs are best tackled with a relatively high, consistent rhythm. So stay planted in the saddle for the majority of it, and sit and spin your way to the top. Give your body mini stretch breaks to keep from tightening up. Periodically, click into a harder gear and stand, pushing your hips forward for low-back relief.

GRIND IT UP THE STEEPS. When the going gets hard, you'll need a low gear, and your cadence will naturally slow down at least a little (likely a lot, if it's *really* steep). Keep your weight evenly distributed over the bike to maintain traction with both tires. (This is especially important if you're off-road on a mountain bike or riding a sketchy unpaved road where your back wheel will slip out faster.) Gently pull through the bars, and press through your legs to power your way up. Stand, as needed, to maintain momentum and keep your head as calm as possible. It may feel like you'll never get over that wall, but you will. Keep your head down and grind it out.

JAM OVER THE CRESTS. When everyone else is sitting up (or slumping forward) at the top of "Heaven's Gate Hill," shift into a higher gear and keep your legs spinning over the other side. You'll not only maintain momentum, but you'll keep your legs fresher for the next climb as you flush out the by-products of your hard work and bring fresh nutrients and oxygenated blood back into your muscle fibers.

4 | BASE CAMP

Your climbing fitness is like a mountain: The broader the base, the higher it can go.

▶ **YOU KNOW WHEN YOU'RE** at a party playing Jenga, and the drunken clown next to you insists on pulling as many pieces from the bottom as he can? While the tower of wooden blocks wobbles and rocks, everyone cringes, waiting for it to come crashing down, because, make no mistake about it, it's going to come crashing down if you keep piling the sticks on top with no support on the bottom. That's a whole lot like how some cyclists (maybe all at one point or another, including yours truly) approach their cycling fitness. They ride hard every time they go out, inevitably crashing and burning, because they haven't built or maintained a rock-solid base.

The key to successful cycling, especially if you're keen to conquer those climbs, is building a solid base of fitness and foundation of strength. This is the platform that lets you stack on higher-intensity rides, efforts, and races without crumbling. When you build a big base, you also push your lactate threshold (LT) higher, effectively building a bigger matchbook, so you can fire off a few when you need them, without panicking like Smokey Bear during a Southern California drought.

There are an awful lot of myths surrounding base training. You've likely heard many of them. Stuff like, "You need to spend months going really slow in your inner chainring to build proper base" or "Intense efforts will wreck your base building." None of that is really true. Here's what good base training is all about, how to build it, and how to build off of it.

ZONE IN

The first step to base training is establishing your training zones. Lots of riders just "ride lots" without putting much thought into how hard (or easy) they're riding. That's obviously A-OK. But, if you want to make measurable gains, especially for challenging rides with lots of climbs, you'll want to divvy up your riding time up into training zones that range from easy like a Sunday morning to ARGH! To monitor your efforts, you can simply use the talk test—when you can talk easily, the effort's easy; when you can barely speak, it's as hard as it gets—but using a training tool like a heart-rate monitor and/or power meter is better, because it keeps you honest and on point. Though pros swear by power training, don't sweat it if you don't want to or can't spring for one. An inexpensive heart-rate monitor will do just fine.

ZONE 1: EASY/RECOVERY

Light, relaxed breathing, barely above normal. You're at 60 to 64 percent of your maximum heart rate (MHR), and less than 55 percent of FTP, if you're using a power meter. You can talk easily. (Rated Perceived Exertion, or RPE, 1 to 2)

ZONE 2: ENDURANCE/BASE

Deep, steady, rhythmic breathing. This is your aerobic, endurance-training zone, requiring 65- to 74-percent MHR (55- to 75-percent FTP). You can speak short sentences but are starting to breathe more heavily. (RPE 3 to 4)

ZONE 3: TEMPO/INTENSIVE ENDURANCE

Slightly labored breathing. This is a steady tempo pace, requiring 75- to 84-percent MHR (75- to 90-percent FTP). You're working just above your endurance comfort zone—similar to when you're riding with someone who is a bit faster than you. You can speak just a few words at a time. (RPE 5 to 6)

ZONE 4: THRESHOLD/ LACTATE THRESHOLD

Short, fast, rhythmic breathing. This is your lactate threshold zone, requiring 85- to 94-percent MHR (90- to 105-percent FTP). You're hitting your sustainable user limit. It's also known as race pace. You can only speak one or two words at a time. (RPE 7 to 8)

ZONE 5: ABOVE THRESHOLD TO MAX

Hard, heavy breathing. This is your VO2 max (the maximum amount of oxygen your body can use; a hallmark of fitness) training zone, where you're at 95- to 100-percent MHR (105- to 120-percent FTP). You're utilizing as much oxygen as possible and going as hard as you can. It is impossible to speak! (RPE 9 to 10)

A CASE TO ACE YOUR BASE

Base training is done at endurance or Zone 2 intensity. Simply put, that's a pace harder than a recovery ride (which should be nearly zero on the effort scale) but not so hard you can't talk the whole time. That talking part? It's key. Because if you can talk, it means that you're using your aerobic energy system, using lots and lots of oxygen to fuel your type I, slow-twitch muscle fibers.

These fibers fuel themselves mostly with stored fat and just a little bit of carbohydrate. Burning fat, of course, is a good thing, because even the wiriest whippets have a nearly infinite supply (and if you're not a wiry whippet, it helps shed unwanted pounds). Type I fibers also are home to the bulk of your muscle's energy-producing mitochondria. When you devote time to building your base, you're stimulating mitochondria growth and improving their function, so you become an even better fat burner. That's particularly useful when you're making your way through the mountains, because your body becomes so good at burning fat that you preserve your precious glycogen (carbohydrate) stores, which gives you the energy you need to go hard at the end of a long, hilly day in the saddle.

Because you're using lots of oxygen during base training, your body adapts to help you get as much oxygen as possible into your working muscles with every heartbeat. That means your heart gets stronger, pumping out more blood per beat, and your body lays down a larger network of capillaries within your muscles, so you can deliver more oxygen and nutrients and carry out more carbon dioxide and metabolic waste products.

The bigger your base, the more metabolic flexibility you have, which is a fancy way of saying that your body gets adept at switching back and forth between fuel sources (carbs and fat), as needed. That has benefits on the bike. Most notably, you'll burn more fat when fuel's running low—a huge help when you're on a long climb with nothing in your jersey pockets but empty sandwich bags.

All of that alone will make you a better climber. But, the metabolic magic of base training doesn't stop there. As mentioned earlier, it also helps raise your threshold, so you can climb at a faster rate of speed before you feel the burn. The secret lies in those hardworking type I fibers.

Your type I, slow-twitch fibers do more than burn fat. They also clear lactate. When you ride harder than your type I muscles can handle, like cranking up a 10-percent climb, your fast-twitch (type II) muscle fibers step in and start blasting glucose from glycogen for energy. The by-product of this process is lactate. We used to think lactate was the enemy of our legs. Now, we know better. Lactate is an essential fuel that your body uses to make energy in your muscles and other cells. What slows you down when you cross that lactate threshold is the hydrogen ions associated with lactate, which can build up and interfere with muscle contraction. To prevent that interference and subsequent slowdown, you need to be able to clear lactate out of your fast-twitch muscles as quickly and efficiently as possible.

That's your type I fibers' job, as was explained to me during an in-depth human performance evaluation by master mitochondria researcher Iñigo San Millán, PhD, of the University of Colorado Sports Medicine and Performance Center in Boulder. These slow-twitch fibers clear lactate through a process called the mitochondrial lactate oxidation complex (mLOC)—which is, as is the case with most cellular metabolism, indeed complex. In short, your fast-twitch fibers shuttle lactate using special transporters called MCT-4. The fuel then hitches a ride into your slow-twitch fibers (which contain the most mitochondria, as well as transporters called MCT-1), where the lactate gets reused for energy. Base training helps your body make more of these transporters and more mitochondria, improving the whole mLOC system, so you can clear lactate faster and go harder for longer without burning up and slowing down.

Sold? Good. Depending on your current state of fitness, it takes 6 to 12 weeks to build a nice solid base. During that time, aim for about 80 percent of your rides to be in those Zone 2 intensities. Once your main riding, racing, and/or event season is in full swing, maintain that base by spending about 40 to 50 percent of your riding time doing long endurance pace rides.

How long do those long base-building rides need to be? People who get paid to ride will be out there pedaling for 5 to 6 hours at a pop. But, that's not realistic or really necessary for riders with day jobs and less free time. A solid base-building ride for most of us is 2 to 3 hours.

That's not to say that there's no room for intensity when you're building your base. There most definitely is, and that's exactly what you should be doing during the rest of your riding time—adding harder efforts. Although some very old-school training dictums (that are really best left to gather dust) say otherwise, the right amount of intensity can help you build your base.

Higher-intensity efforts trigger those type II turbo fibers, which you need to build your top end and can produce some aerobic, fat-burning benefits of their own, according to a growing body of research on high-intensity interval training (HIIT). It all comes back to the mighty mitochondria, says HIIT proponent Paul Laursen, PhD, an exercise

HOW DO YOU KNOW WHEN YOU'VE BUILT YOUR BASE?

If you keep a training log or use a service like Strava, you can track your performance. Or, you can go by intuition. On rides in similar and not extreme conditions, the speed of your Zone 2 endurance rides should improve, and those rides should feel easier. When you feel like you've hit a plateau and you're not making any more measurable gains, you've pretty much built your base. If you use a power meter and heart-rate monitor, you can get more scientific about it by dividing your average power output for your endurance rides by your average heart rate for the same rides. This is what TrainingPeaks software calls your efficiency factor. During base building, that number should trend upward. When it stabilizes, your base is built.

physiologist with the training service PlewsandProf.com.

"Ultimately, your 'base' comes down to your mitochondrial capacity," he says. "While longer, lower-intensity exercise increases the number of mitochondria in your cells, high-intensity training makes those mitochondria more powerful." Some studies show that high-intensity exercise performed regularly can stimulate the production of mitochondria, as well.

What's more, when you do high-intensity intervals, your heart rate stays elevated during your recovery periods, so you're still tapping into and developing your aerobic energy system. Even really fit cyclists get an endurance performance bump, says Dr. Laursen. "We found that when well-trained cyclists performed two interval sessions a week for 3 to 6 weeks, their VO_2 max peak aerobic-power output and endurance performance improved by 2 to 4 percent."

RAISE YOUR ROOF

To build upon your base and make your way up the mountains faster, you need to add intervals—all kinds of intervals, but most specifically those that will raise your lactate threshold as high as possible, so you can produce more power at a comfortable heart rate. To accomplish that, when you're not doing recovery or Zone 2 endurance rides, you should be doing rides that include high and very high intensities, hitting a blend of zones 3 to 5 throughout the week. These not only help raise your threshold but also boost endurance.

Dr. Laursen is partial to relatively short, very hard intervals of 30 seconds to 5 minutes. These build your aerobic system and are also hard enough to recruit some fast-twitch sprint fibers, which makes those power-producing fibers more resistant to fatigue over time. "Performing three to six of these leg-burning efforts, allowing 1 to 2 minutes of recovery in between, can have impressive effects," he says.

But, those aren't the only intervals to include in your hill-climbing arsenal. Others are just as important and add variety to your cycling repertoire.

Below, you'll find a selection of some key workouts. Aim to perform one of these interval sessions twice a week, allowing at least a day of recovery in between. (For a complete training plan that pulls together riding and off-the-bike workouts, see Chapter 12.)

STEADY-STATE INTERVALS

Probably the most effective way to increase your power at threshold is to perform long, steady intervals where you hover just below your threshold (see "Your LT Field Test" on page 44). They're relatively easy to do, but require concentration, because it can be easy to let your mind (and your effort) drift.

DO IT: After a 10- to 15-minute warm-up (zones 1 to 2), ride 10 minutes at a steady effort, keeping your heart rate three to five beats below your LT heart rate (Zone 3/RPE 6). Recover for 5 to 10 minutes (you're aiming for adequate recovery, so you can maintain your targeted intensity for the next effort), then repeat two more times. Once those feel easy, do two 20-minute steady-state efforts, recovering for 10 to 20 minutes between. Eventually, work up to one 30-minute effort.

🎯 YOUR LT FIELD TEST

The most precise way to find your lactate threshold (LT) is in a lab, where you pedal at increasingly hard intensities, while a technician draws blood and checks your levels. (There also are optical sensors you can wear on your calf that are quite accurate.) But, you can get a good estimate yourself by performing a field test.

Map a 3-mile route that you can ride without stopping. Strap on a heart-rate monitor, warm up for 20 minutes, then ride the route at the fastest pace you can sustain. Recover for 10 to 20 minutes (ride back to the start of your route at an easy pace). Repeat the test. Your LT is approximately the average heart rate of the two efforts. (More accurately, it's 103 percent of that figure.) Jot down your times and average paces; repeat the test in 8 weeks to see your progress.

You can also replicate the test on an indoor trainer by pedaling the fastest pace you can sustain for 20 to 30 minutes (after a good warm-up, of course). Your average heart rate over the duration is roughly your lactate threshold. If you have a power meter, you can use the same test to determine your functional threshold power or FTP, a metric that represents the highest power output you can sustain for about 1 hour, which has been championed by power-training gurus Hunter Allen and Dr. Andy Coggan, co-authors of *Training and Racing with a Power Meter*, and Joe Friel, creator of *The Cyclist's Training Bible*. Your FTP would be 95 percent of your average power over that 20-minute period. FTP is also a good marker of climbing success and useful for tracking your progress.

TOLERANCE (AKA SUFFERING THRESHOLD) INTERVALS

Obviously, climbing in the real world is not steady. You're going to be forced into the red sometimes, especially if you're trying to keep up with others or shooting for a personal best or race finish. That means you need to train your body to quickly recover from pushing into the red, as well as improving your ability to tolerate crossing that threshold. These two intervals will help pave the way.

UP AND DOWNS

These intervals blend LT and VO2 max (your body's ability to process oxygen) training (zones 4 and 5) to simulate the effort you need when pushing hard over hilly terrain.

DO IT: Warm up, as needed. Then pick up the pace until you reach your LT heart rate (Zone 4/RPE 8), and hold that intensity for 5 to 6 minutes. Then, increase your effort to three to five beats above LT (low Zone 5/RPE 9) for 1 to 2 minutes. Then, drop it back down to LT. Continue this way for a total of three cycles, or about 20 minutes.

EXTENDED BURSTS

These above-LT efforts boost your ability to keep riding hard in the face of high-lactate levels, which is helpful for staying strong over punchy terrain.

DO IT: Warm up, as needed. Increase your effort to about five beats above your LT heart rate (low Zone 5/RPE 9). Hold it there for 2 to 3 minutes. Reduce your effort to easy (Zone 1/RPE 2) for half the interval time, 60 to 90 seconds, just long enough so you feel partially recovered but not quite ready to go again. And, then, go again! Repeat three times.

CLIMBING INTERVALS

No-brainer: If you want to get better at climbing, you climb! You can do hill repeats, which as the name implies, means going up and down the same hill multiple times. Or, just map out a hilly route. Ideally, find a climb that lets you pedal at or near your threshold (Zone 4/RPE 7 to 8) for at least 10 minutes, up to 30 is even better.

Every few minutes, click into a harder gear, get out of the saddle, and go harder (Zone 5) for 10 to 20 pedal strokes.

WHAT IF YOU DON'T HAVE HILLS?

Are you hopelessly screwed if you want to do hilly events but don't live near many climbs? Nope. Though it would behoove you to take a few trips to train in bumpy terrain ahead of time, you can make the metabolic gains you need to no matter where you live. Excellent case in point is coach Ian Marling, of Bell Lap Coaching in Massachusetts, who has steadily improved his time up Mount Washington in New Hampshire from 1:32 to 1:14—an enormous gain on a 7.6-mile climb. His secret weapon: Time trialing.

"Preparing for Mount Washington, I didn't do a lot of training on specific climbs," he says. "I just found an 8-mile route and rode that thing flat out. Metabolically, it's the same level of effort as a long climb. I would also do multi-zone efforts where I would do a tempo [Zone 3] ride and throw VO2 max [Zone 5] bursts into it. You can do that on a perfectly flat road. That kind of changing effort from hard to harder to hardest and back down mimics what you need to do to get to the top of a hard climb."

Other flatlanders who raced Mount Washington shared similar training techniques, including women's record-setter Victoria Di Savino, of Buffalo. "I work long hours, so I don't have the opportunity to travel to the hills to train," she says. "I just go out and do three 20-minute efforts at threshold, which is pretty much the equivalent of the power you use to go up Mount Washington."

Bonus points if you can do these efforts into the wind, says Jonathan Simmons, another Mount Washington aficionado who lives on the decidedly flat Cape Cod. "I go out on the Cape Cod Canal and do my 20-minute intervals going into a 20-mph headwind. It's what my Dutch friends would call climbing the Alps of Holland!"

BUILD A SOLID FRAME—YOURS

An all-too-often overlooked element of building base and a strong foundation is core training. You can have legs as strong as redwoods, but if your core is as wobbly as a willow in the wind, you're going to be wasting watts because when your core gets weak, you transfer less power from your upper body to your lower body. That makes you less stable in the saddle and unable to push maximum power into your pedals. It also leaves you vulnerable to tight, achy back muscles, which will most definitely slow you down. Strong core muscles increase your power transfer from your arms to your legs, especially when you're pushing out of the saddle. The stronger you get, the bigger the gear you can push up hills and the faster you can reach the top.

For climbing purposes, you want to hit your entire core, which includes your back, abs, sides, and hips (your core doesn't stop where your jeans begin). The moves on pages 48 to 54 will get it done. Perform the routine as a circuit: Do 10 to 15 reps of each exercise, moving immediately from exercise to exercise, without rest. When you're finished, rest a minute, if you need to, and repeat the sequence once. Aim to work your core 2 to 3 days a week—even during riding season.

TIPPING BIRD

I love this move for targeting the hips and glutes, which can be notoriously weak in cyclists. Because you work one leg at a time, it also helps even out common imbalances.

DO IT: Stand tall with your arms out to the side at shoulder height. Keeping your left leg extended, lift your left foot behind you and balance on your right leg. Slowly hinge forward from the hips, tipping your torso forward toward the ground, while extending your left leg straight behind you, foot flexed, until your body forms a straight line from your head to your heel. Stop when you're parallel to the floor. Return to start, and repeat on the other side—that's one rep.

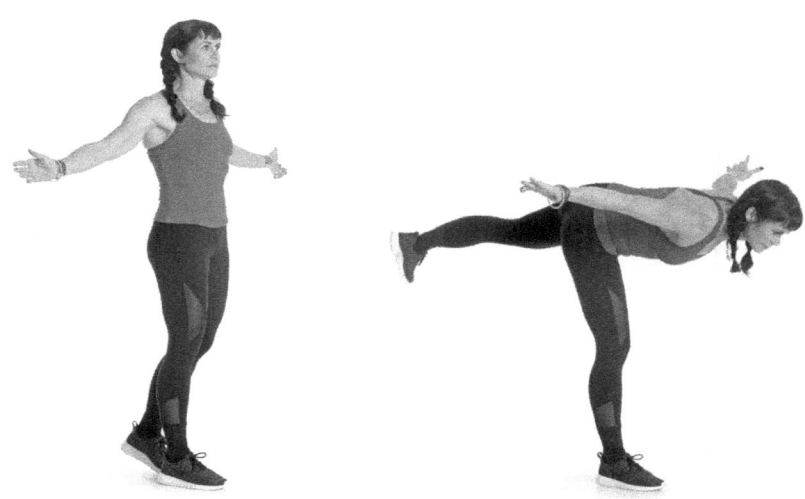

TT PLANK

Planks are a climber's best friend, because they strengthen all those core muscles that help keep your upper body quiet while your legs are doing the talking up the mountainside. There are countless variations, but this one is particularly good if you do triathlons or time trials, because it puts your arms in the same position that you'll be in on your aero bars.

DO IT: Keeping your elbows on the floor directly beneath your shoulders, forearms extended and hands in loose fists, lift your body into a plank pose, resting on your toes and maintaining a neutral spine. Hold for 20 to 30 seconds, gradually building up to a minute or even 2, if you're a long-distance rider.

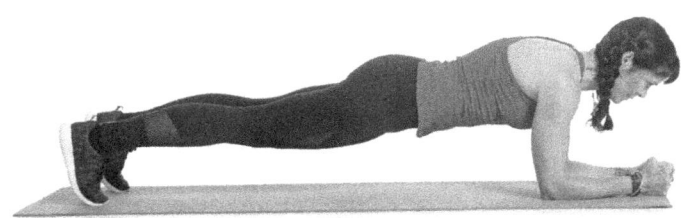

COBRA LIFT

We cyclists spend a lot of time flexed forward. If you work a desk job, you likely spend the lion's share of your waking hours in that forward keyboard slump. This move tones and strengthens your stretched-out and often weak flip side by strengthening the erector spinae, lumbar, and glute muscles.

DO IT: Lie face-down, legs extended, arms out and back about 45 degrees, palms down. Contract your glutes, squeeze your shoulder blades together, press your legs into the floor, and lift as much of your torso up off the floor as far as you can (this may be just your chest), rotating your arms so your thumbs point to the ceiling. Keep your neck straight. Pause. Return to start position.

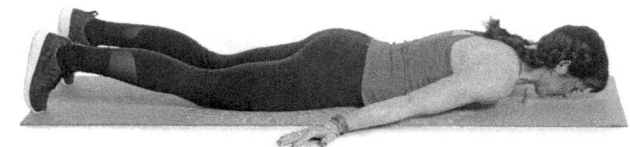

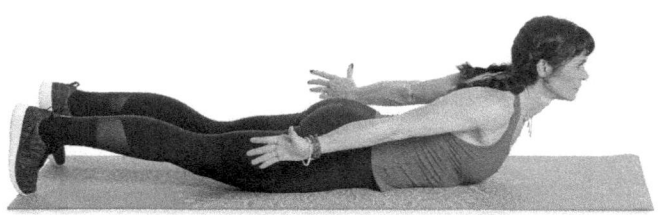

SCORPION

Cyclists often have weak hips and lumbar (back) muscles, and those muscles can also get tight, limiting your mobility on and off the bike. This fierce core move strengthens your lumbar and glute muscles and improves mobility and range of motion throughout your pelvic girdle (the area that connects your torso to your legs). As a nice bonus, it stretches your chest, hips, shoulders, and back.

DO IT: Lie face-down with your arms out to the sides (straight or bent, whichever is most comfortable), shoulders flat on the floor. Bend your left leg 90 degrees, then lift it off the floor. Twisting your torso, bring that leg across the back of your body as far as possible—try to touch the floor with your foot under your right hand. Return to start. Then, repeat on the other side. That's one rep.

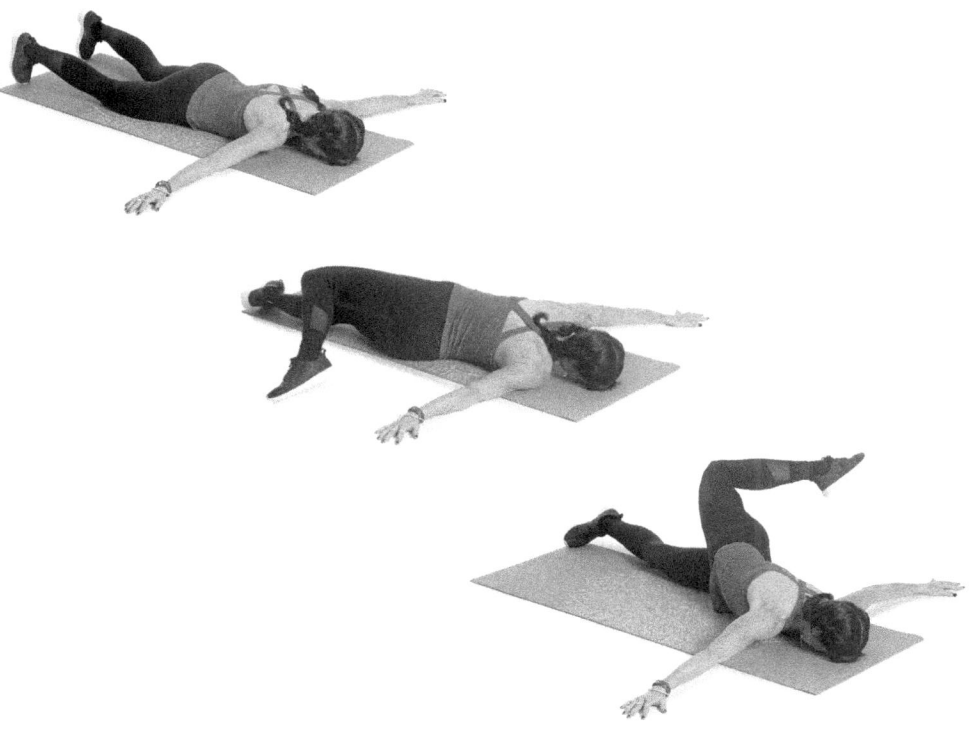

BRIDGE

Hey, look, another move for your glutes and lower back (sensing a trend?). Bridges hone in on the muscles where your lower back meets the top of your glutes, a spot where cyclists often get achy when they climb.

DO IT: Lying on your back, with your knees bent and your feet flat on the floor, squeeze your glutes and raise your hips toward the ceiling so your body forms a straight line from your shoulders to your knees. Pause. Then, lower to the floor and repeat. When that gets easy, lift one leg off the floor to do single-leg bridges.

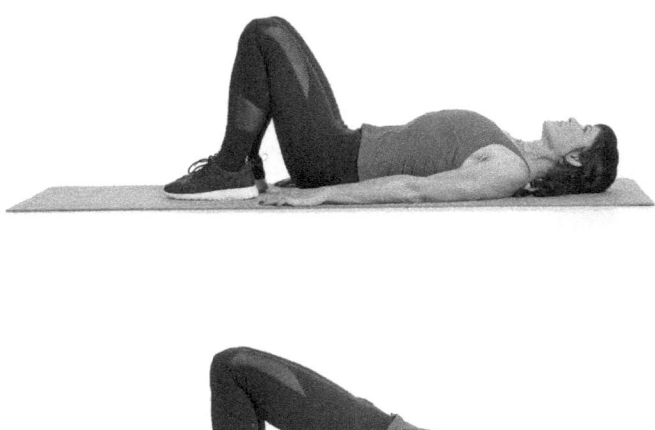

RUSSIAN TWIST

This rotational move is great for building strong obliques, as well as your deep transverse abdominal muscles, which are key for stabilizing your torso when you're climbing.

DO IT: Hold a medicine ball (or dumbbell by the ends) in both hands. Sit on the floor with your knees bent, feet flat on the floor. Keeping your back straight, lean back slightly and lift your feet slightly off the ground (it looks like the boat pose in yoga). Twist your torso all the way to one side, then all the way to the other. Keep your neck and shoulders relaxed. Do 10 to 15 reps on each side. To make it harder, lean back farther.

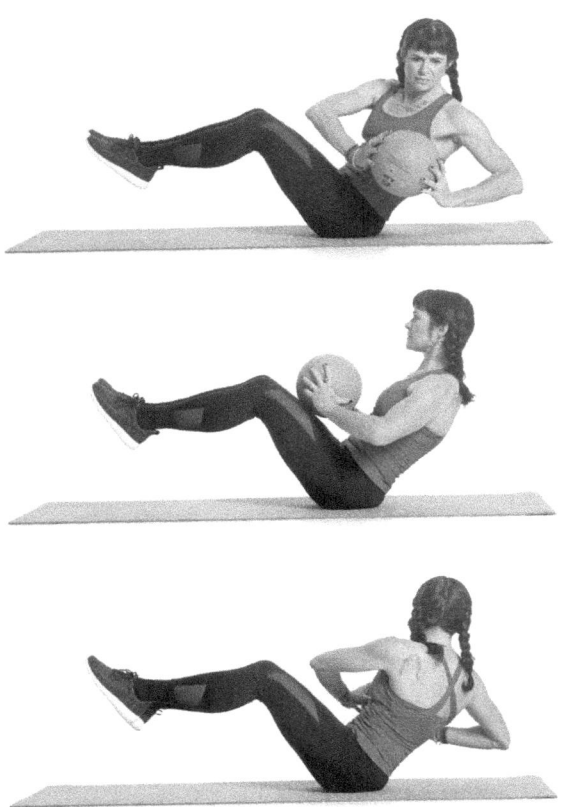

BALL PIKE

If you don't have a stability ball, it's totally worth buying one to take your core work to the next level by doing moves such as this one. Because you're on an unstable platform, your entire core has to fire up to keep you steady—ideal for building core stability for riding a bike.

DO IT: Start in a plank position with your hands on the floor, your arms extended (as they'd be at the top of a push-up), and the tops of your feet up on an inflated stability ball. Keeping your knees straight, hike your hips toward the ceiling, so your back is straight and your butt is pointed up toward the ceiling. Lower to the plank position and repeat. If that's too tough, do stability ball tucks: From the start position, bend your knees and pull the ball in toward your chest.

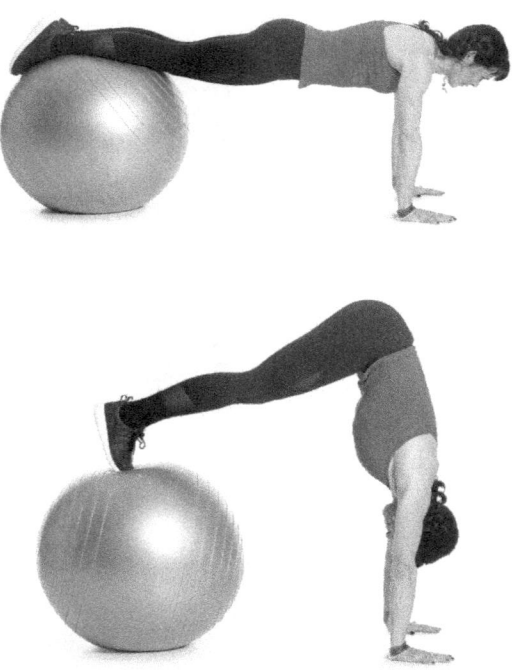

ON-BIKE CORE CONDITIONING

You can complement your off-bike core training with strengthening exercises you can do while you ride. Here's a low-cadence climbing exercise for you to toss into the mix once or twice a week.

Warm up for 10 to 15 minutes, then head to a moderate climb (5- to 8-percent grade) and perform 2-minute seated, low-cadence climbing efforts. To do it, simply keep your bike in a bigger-than-normal gear and push smooth, hard pedal strokes at 50 to 60 rpm. Your cadence should still be fluid, just slower and more forceful—but it shouldn't be so slow and difficult that you're rocking back and forth on the bike or mashing on the pedals. Recover for 1 to 2 minutes, and repeat to the top of the climb, or four or five more times. This helps build hip as well as knee strength and makes your muscles and connective tissue more resilient.

5 YOUR POWER STATION

All the ways you can produce more watts.

▶ **THE FIRST WORD IN** the power-to-weight equation is power—the rate at which you can do work (produce watts), or work divided by time. Simply put, the more watts you can throw down when the road tilts up, the faster you can make it to the top. We'll take a crack at achieving optimum weight in Chapter 8. But, first things first: This chapter (which assumes you've dutifully built your base—see Chapter 4) is devoted to the best ways to build mountain-smashing wattage.

GET STRONG

Strength is the foundation of power, and the foundation of strength is muscle-fiber development—i.e., strength training. If you're one of those cyclists who neglects or resists strength training because you don't think it's important—or worse, think it's counterproductive, think again. Strength training is not about bodybuilding or getting huge muscles. Done properly, it increases your watts without weighing you down by improving the following:

YOUR NEURAL DRIVE: This is your mind-muscle connection, which stimulates muscle contraction. Your muscle fibers are bundled into motor units, which are activated by your brain when you need to do a job. When you start challenging your muscles through strength training, your brain goes, "Whoa, we need more muscle power!" and activates more units. Those neuromuscular connections are then at your disposal on your bike. So, if you've never busted out a squat, you can see gains nearly instantly through this stimulus alone.

YOUR CAPACITY: The more muscle fibers you train, the more you can recruit to help you up a climb. Strength training makes your fast-twitch type II fibers more fatigue resistant, so they can hammer harder longer and stiffen your tendons for greater stability in the saddle. Both are essential for successful climbing.

YOUR EFFICIENCY: This is a biggie and largely overlooked. When you combine the first two benefits (above), you improve your neuromuscular efficiency, which is a fancy way of saying that your brain can quickly recruit all the muscles you need to push your pedals.

Contrary to old-school thinking that strength training impedes cycling performance, a growing body of research shows that endurance athletes who include heavy and/or explosive strength training in their routines significantly improve their max power, efficiency, economy and their time-trial performance over those who stick to strictly endurance work.

This is especially important as we age, because we naturally start to lose muscle mass after age 30. It's even more important for women, who have less muscle mass to begin with. But, that's not to say that everyone, including uberfit young cyclists, can't benefit from dedicated strength training. Today's generation of elite pros—yes, even the Kings of the Mountains like Joe Dombrowski and Alex Howes—swear by strength training.

"My favorite two moves in the gym are squats and deadlifts," says Howes. "When done properly, they hit every muscle that matters in the lower body and really strengthen the muscles in the lower back, which are key to good form and power transfer on the bike." Howes also appreciates how strength training makes him feel rock solid in the saddle, so the power he puts into his pedals propels him uphill with fewer wasted watts.

Dombrowski adds a leg press into the mix. "I focus on three big moves: squat, deadlift, and leg press, in that order. I often am doing them to failure, so it's best to finish with the safest move, as you're more fatigued," says the climbing specialist, who credits the routine with helping him gain functional muscle mass in the off-season, as well as maintain good form during the season.

HOW TO GET IT DONE

Most cyclists want stronger, but not necessarily bigger, muscles. That means lifting fewer repetitions of heavier weight. For the exercises that follow, you should use weight that you cannot lift more than five times. For instance, you could perform five sets of five reps or four sets of three or four reps of close-to-your-max weight,* with generous amounts of recovery (about 4 minutes) between sets. This type of lifting stimulates your neural drive, improves your intramuscular coordination (so the fibers in any given muscle work better in concert to generate force), stimulates growth-hormone production, and generates myofibrillar hypertrophy, which means that your muscle fibers become denser and stronger, but not necessarily larger (i.e., sarcoplasmic hypertrophy), which is exactly what cyclists—especially climbers—need.

If you already lift weights, you can transition to heavy, low-rep lifting to bust through a plateau and enjoy strength gains. If you're new to strength training, you will need to lift lighter weights with higher reps (i.e., two or

---

*To determine your max weight (known as one-rep max), warm up with 12 to 15 reps of very light weight. Then, slowly increase the weights until you can perform just one rep with perfect form. That's your one-rep max.

three sets of 10 to 12 reps) for 3 or 4 months to become comfortable executing the exercises with proper form and to condition your connective tissues to tolerate heavier work.

How do you fit this into your riding schedule? As with all training, everyone responds differently, so you may need to do a little trial and error. In general, when you're riding less, like in the winter, you can easily lift more often—say 2 or 3 days a week. When you're riding more, you can go into maintenance mode and lift once a week. One time-efficient way to work in weights is to piggyback your resistance training with your interval rides. So, warm up with your weight workout, then bang out your hard ride. That way, you can recover from both training stimuli on your recovery or rest day the following day.

SQUAT

Stand with your feet hip-width to shoulder-width apart and your toes pointed slightly out. Hold dumbbells at your shoulders or down at your sides. Push your butt and hips back as if you were sitting in a chair and lower down as far as possible, while keeping your weight on your heels. Return to the starting position and repeat.

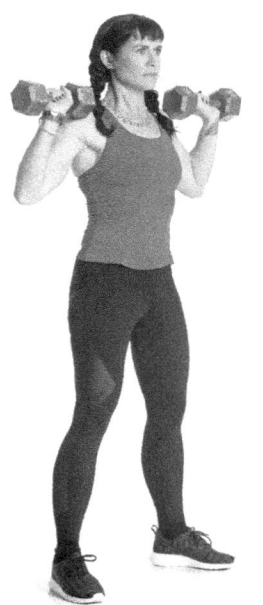
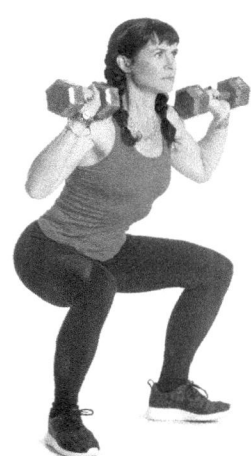

DEADLIFT

Hold a barbell in front of your thighs, arms extended, palms facing in. Keep your back flat. Hinge at the hips and lower the weight toward the floor, allowing your knees to bend slightly. Keep the weight close to your body and lower it until your upper body is almost parallel to the floor. Contracting your glutes, push your hips forward to raise yourself back to the starting position.

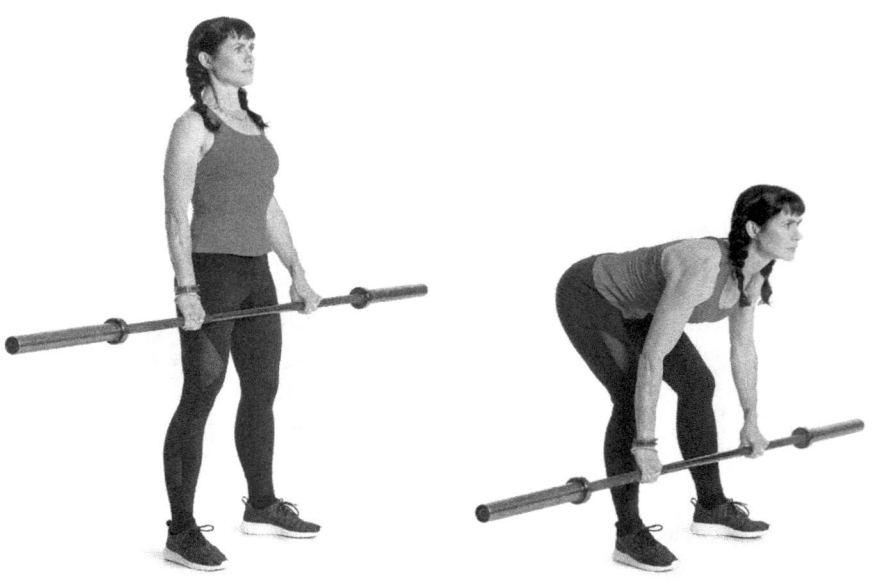

LEG PRESS

Sit on a leg press machine with your feet pressed against the footplate about the same distance apart as they are on the bike, knees bent. Holding the handles on either side, extend your legs and push the weight up and away, keeping your feet flat. Don't lock your knees. Slowly let your legs relax and drop back toward you, bending your knees back to start position. Repeat.

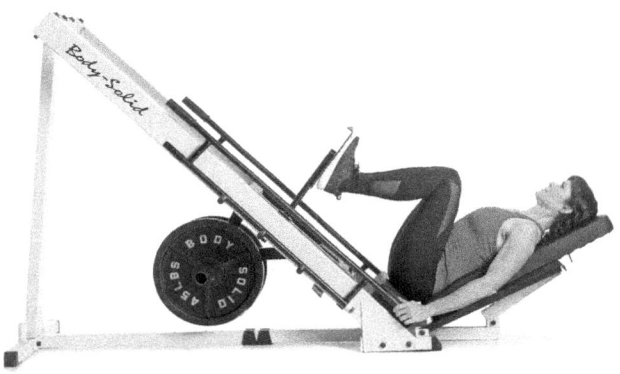

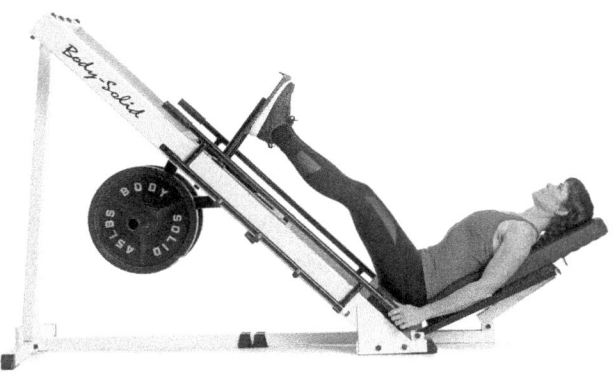

EXPLODE UPHILL

To build the explosive power and force production (the ability to produce a high amount of power in a short amount of time) you need to conquer punchy climbs, surge through switchbacks, and jump when your riding buddies attack on the uphill, add some plyometrics—explosive moves that are performed by loading up a muscle and contracting it rapidly—to the mix. These are especially useful if you find yourself getting dropped on the climby sections of crit or cyclocross courses, says Kerry Werner, a rider on the Kona Endurance and Adventure Team. Werner does Olympic style power-lifting, including the squats and deadlifts above, as well as plyometrics.

"I do explosive lifting and plyometric jumping moves like box jumps, both double- and single-legged," he says. "My goal is to help my muscles adapt so that they can generate and tolerate lots of snap. It also improves my stability on the bike, by adding another dimension of movement besides the up and down of cycling."

Research shows that when cyclists add high-resistance training and plyometrics to their routine, they can make major gains in sprint and endurance performance in just 4 to 5 weeks. I really appreciate how plyometrics improve my ability to climb technical terrain on my mountain bike.

These moves can be tacked onto your strength-training workout or done in place of them, to stimulate your muscles in novel ways.

HOW IT'S DONE

Before starting plyometrics, you should have at least a month of strength-training (like squats and deadlifts) under your belt. Proper form and technique is essential. Warm up thoroughly. Always land softly by recoiling your joints like a spring immediately as you hit the ground.

BOX JUMPS

Stand facing a 12- to 18-inch-high box or step. Squat down and jump up using a double arm swing. Land firmly on the box with your knees soft, to absorb impact. Step down, and repeat. When you've mastered that, try adding a set of one-legged jumps (using a lower box or step to start). Aim for 8 to 12 reps, but perform only as many reps as you can with proper form.

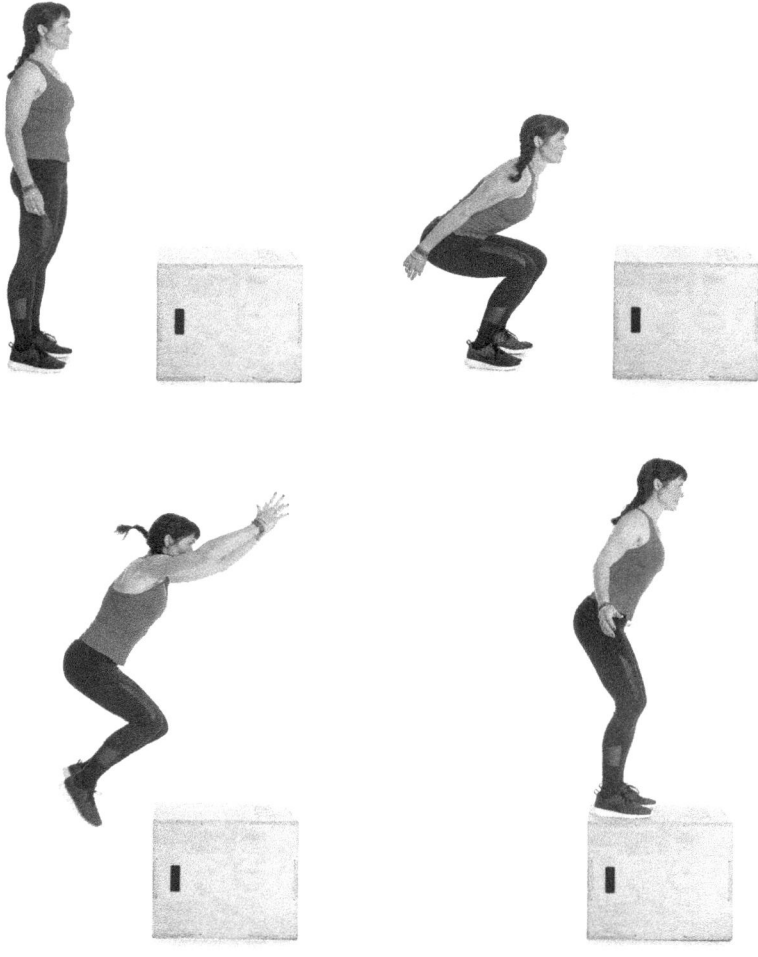

WEIGHTED JUMP SQUATS

Hold a pair of dumbbells that are about 25 percent of your max squat weight (combined—start with lighter weight to perfect form), arms extended down at your sides. Stand with your feet hip-width apart. Bend your hips and knees to squat down until your legs are bent at 90 degrees. Immediately jump explosively into the air. Land softly and immediately drop into the next squat jump. Aim to perform five to eight reps.

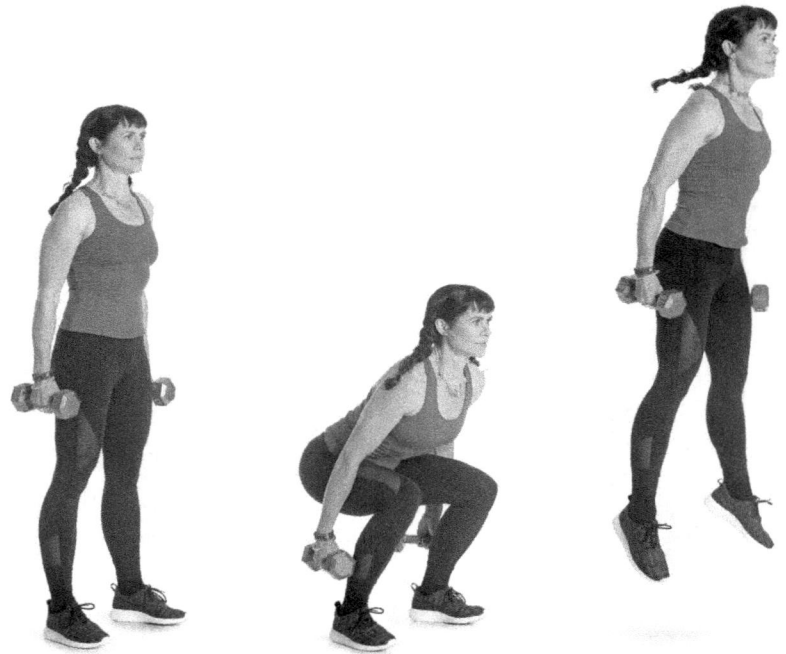

BRING IT BACK TO THE BIKE

To convert your newfound strength into on-the-bike speed, get on the bike and throw down some watts with high-intensity interval training (HIIT). When you push yourself to your absolute upper limits, everything, including endurance, lactate threshold, efficiency, and, of course, power and speed—comes along for the ride, even in well-trained cyclists. In a study of 38 conditioned riders, Australian researchers found that those doing high-intensity interval training twice a week slashed their 40K time-trial time by nearly 3 minutes (about 5 percent) and improved their average speed by nearly 1 mile per hour.

Big climbing bonus: Study author and endurance coach Paul Laursen, PhD, adjunct professor of exercise physiology at Auckland University of Technology, noted that this type of interval training also appears to make your fast-twitch fibers more fatigue resistant, so they behave more like slow-twitch fibers, allowing you to climb at a quick clip even longer.

Here are the best short workouts for all your climbing needs (many of them don't even require a hill). For each interval session, warm up for at 5 to 10 minutes. Cool down, as needed, when you're done. Rotate through these as you like (so you're doing just one type of interval per session) during your weekly workouts. Do these no more than twice a week, preferably midweek, if you're riding long and/or hard on the weekends. You'll see improvements in just 2 weeks.

FAST-ACTING TABATA INTERVALS

Named after the now-famous Japanese exercise scientist Izumi Tabata, these eye-popping efforts train your body to recruit maximum muscle fibers and fire them faster, as well as raise your lactate threshold and, therefore, your climbing prowess.

DO IT: After a warm-up, sprint as hard as possible (Zone 5; you're going for maximum wattage) for 20 seconds. Stop and coast for just 10 seconds. Repeat six to eight times. Rest for 5 minutes. Repeat two or three more times.

PUNCHY UPS

These slightly longer micro-intervals build power and train your body to recover quickly between hard pushes. You'll appreciate these intervals if you ride with a group that likes to push the pace on climbs.

DO IT: In a medium to big gear, push as hard as you can (Zone 5) for 40 seconds. Recover for 20 seconds. Repeat 10 times. Rest for 5 minutes. Do two or three more sets.

FULL-RECOVERY FULL THROTTLES

These max-effort intervals allow complete recovery in between efforts so that you can maintain full intensity for each interval without a drop in power. These mimic the type of effort you need for hilly rides, where you're charging up and over a series of short, spread-out hills.

DO IT: Warm up, then do 30 seconds all-out (Zone 5) followed by 4:30 minutes of easy spinning; then 20 seconds all-out, 4:45 minutes easy; 10 seconds all-out, 5:00 minutes easy. Repeat the whole sequence two more times.

HILL CHARGES

There are times when you need a bit of turbo boost to power through a steep switchback, crest a climb without getting dropped, or beat your buddies to the top. These max-effort drills accomplish that.

DO IT: Climb at a pace that is just about threshold (Zone 4/RPE 8 to 9). When you're ready, attack and push as hard as you can (Zone 5) for 10 to 20 pedal strokes (about 10 to 20 seconds). Back down to threshold or a bit below for 10 to 20 seconds. Repeat four more times. Spin easy for 10 minutes and repeat the intervals from the top, if you're so inclined.

POWER SURGES

The punchy nature of climbs often pops riders because it forces them into the red without adequate recovery. This interval helps to develop more power at your threshold, so you'll be better conditioned to handle changes in pitch and intensity.

DO IT: Start climbing at an intensity that is just under your threshold (Zone 3/RPE 6). After 3 minutes, push your pace/intensity so that you're right at threshold (Zone 4/RPE 7 to 8). After 2 minutes, push your pace so that you're above threshold (Zone 5/ RPE 9). Hold for 1 minute. Recover for 5 to 6 minutes. Repeat for a total of two or three surges.

BIG GEAR ACCELERATION

These drills are a great way for flatlanders to improve their power on climbs.

DO IT: On a straight, flat, open road, shift into bigger gears until you come to a slow roll (between 5 and 10 mph). From a seated position, push the pace as hard as you can (Zone 5) for 10 to 12 seconds. Recover for 60 seconds. Repeat for a total of five surges. You can do one or two sets of these within a ride—just give yourself at least 30 minutes recovery between sets.

RAMPS

Sustainable power is where it's at, if you want to PR (or just survive, depending on the circumstances!) on long climbs. Progressive ramped intervals that start fairly easy and end hard are a great way to raise your functional threshold power and psychologically prepare you for the rigors of seemingly endless ascents. Perform these intervals 2 x 20-style (two efforts for 20 minutes, with 10 minutes recovery between efforts).

DO IT: Start at the lower end of your threshold (Zone 4/RPE 7). Hold it there for about 10 minutes. Then, push the effort to the upper end of your threshold (Zone 4/RPE 8) and hold for about 8 minutes. Finish by notching it up to close to your max (Zone 5/RPE 9) for the final 2 minutes of the interval.

For a complete training plan that pulls together the riding and off-the-bike training, see Chapter 10.

RECOVER RIGHT

Training hard and digging deep will make you strong enough to dance up mountainsides only if you also make the effort to help your body to recover, so it has what it needs to rebuild. Otherwise, instead of standing on a summit above the tree line soaking in the magnificent views, you'll find yourself barely able to climb your stairs at home, wondering what went wrong.

Fitness gains from hard efforts work like this: You saddle up and throttle yourself with threshold ramps and hill repeats, maybe some box jumps, and after you rack your bike and hit the showers, your body goes, "OMG! That was ridiculous. We better bolster up the power and energy systems around here lest that psycho wants to do that again!" And, your body gets to work, repairing damaged muscles and building a stronger muscular system; shuttling out the metabolic waste and bringing in fresh blood and oxygen; restocking and replenishing your fuel, electrolyte, and hydration stores; and shifting your body from a state of fight or flight into rest and digest, so you can get fired up again without feeling burned out.

That takes time. You need 24 to 48 hours, at least, for your muscles to recover from tough efforts—whether extremely hard or very long—that leave them tapped out. Full-muscle recovery is important not only because recovered muscles are stronger and less sore but also because they're better able to fully store glycogen, which is essential to power you up and over the next hill . . . and the one after that . . . and the one after that.

How long your mind needs to recover is less quantifiable. But, since your brain and body operate on a continuous feedback loop, anything you do to facilitate physical recovery will help your mental state as well, and vice versa.

The science of recovery is constantly evolving, but there are a few constants that you can count on to get all your systems back to "go" after a hard day (or series of days) has them moving slowly. Here's what works.

PREGAME THE RECOVERY PROCESS. The word "recovery" implies post-exercise, but having a protein-rich snack beforehand will minimize muscle damage and hasten the rebuilding process before you even click in. "Aim to get 15 to 20 grams of protein before hard efforts," says exercise physiologist Stacy Sims, PhD, senior research fellow at the Adams High Performance Centre at the University of Waikato in New Zealand. She recommends eating Greek yogurt, which serves up 15 grams of protein in just 6 ounces and provides the amino acid leucine, which is key for building muscle.

FLICK THE RECOVERY SWITCH IMMEDIATELY AFTER. Your body goes into a catabolic state—basically eating into its own muscles—after exhausting efforts. Priority one is flipping that state to become anabolic (building up rather than breaking down muscle tissue). That means pumping in some protein within 30 minutes of finishing, if possible. That's especially important for women, because female hormones tend to leave women more catabolic than men. Include some carbohydrates to restock your glycogen stores. Nutritionists like Dina Griffin, RD, CSSD, CISSN, performance education coordinator at eNRG Performance in Littleton, Colorado, recommend aiming for a post-ride snack that comprises 15 to 25 grams of protein and 15 to 30 grams of carbohydrate. A cup of Greek yogurt with ¼ cup granola will get you there.

ICE, ICE, MAYBE: Whenever I raced with multitime world champion mountain biker Rebecca Rusch, she would just about force me into an ice bath or freezing cold stream or lake afterward, which I loathed but always did, because she's Rebecca Rusch and I'm not. Left to my own accord, I'd skip the icy plunge. And as it turns out, neither of us is necessarily right or wrong. Ice baths are a long-standing recovery technique designed to trick your body into redistributing the blood from your still-warm skin back into central circulation to shuttle out metabolic waste, as well as to decrease swelling and inflammation in your muscles.

But, studies on their actual effectiveness are equivocal, with some suggesting ice baths alone may actually delay recovery. What may work better when you're in a bad way is contrast therapy, where you alternate cold and heat to passively push and pull blood in and out of your muscles. In one study, exercisers who received contrast therapy after shredding their legs on the leg press machine enjoyed faster recovery of their strength and power than their peers who just rested afterward. Don't happen to have an ice tub and Jacuzzi in your house? Take a contrast shower—alternating hot and cold temperatures during your post-ride clean-up. Or, fake it with ice packs (or bags of frozen peas) and hot-water bottles, applying the cold packs to your worked-over quads for about 5 minutes, followed by the hot-water bottles, and so forth for two to three cycles.

REST UP. There's a saying that races are won in bed, which is to say that sleep is essential for full recovery. As you slumber, your body pumps out human growth hormone, which is responsible for tissue growth and repair. If possible, sneak in 40 winks during the day, as well, especially after particularly grueling efforts. Research shows that a daytime power nap about 2 hours after a hard effort helps your body slip into a deep, restorative state of sleep. Naps are particularly potent when you're not sleeping your best, like when traveling for an event. A study in the *Journal of Clinical Endocrinology and Metabolism* reports that just 30 minutes of stolen shuteye is enough to restore stress hormones and immunity to normal levels after a night of short sleep.

SPIN IT OUT. You may not feel like leaving your recliner the day after a hard, hilly century or otherwise shredding effort, but your legs will thank you if you get up and get the lead out. You'll recover more quickly than if you sit around. (Spinning also works better than stretching, which feels good but doesn't really speed recovery.) In a study that compared passive recovery (i.e., sitting on your rump, remote in hand), stretching, and active recovery (cycling with minimal resistance), following a fatiguing bout of exercise, those who pedaled easy recovered far better than those in the other two groups, who saw little improvement. Just be sure to not overdo it. Your ride should be no more strenuous than a stroll through the neighborhood.

FLUSH THE SYSTEM. In a perfect world, we'd all have a massage therapist waiting for us, fuzzy robe in hand, to flush out our tattered quads and calves after a hard day on the bike. The world is an imperfect place. But, it's still worthwhile flushing your muscles any way you can, to remove the metabolic waste and revive them with fresh nutrient and oxygen-rich blood, which is key to recovery. You can go high tech with specific recovery devices such as compression pumps, like Elevated Legs (inflated leg sleeves that use pneumatic compression to enhance bloodflow), or an electrical stimulation device, like Marc Pro, which makes your muscles contract via electrodes, literally without you moving a muscle. You can treat yourself to a regular sports massage. You also can go old school and use self-massage tools like the Stick, ROLL Recovery, and/or foam rollers.

CHILL OUT. Exercise is a form of stress. Much of life is another form of stress. The latter can impede your recovery from the former, by keeping you in a state of fight or flight. Practice a relaxation technique like deep breathing. Simply inhale deeply through your nose and into your lungs, expanding your diaphragm to a count of three or four; then exhale for a count of three or four, and repeat for a few cycles. Research shows this type of systematic, controlled breathing is a powerful nervous-system calmer.

6 | F%CK!

How to stay calm and climb on.

▶ **CLIMBING. AT ITS ESSENCE,** is a mental undertaking—one where your mind can play tricks and the elevation of OMG! is often inversely related to the elevation of the climb, as evidenced in the flowchart on page 76.

There are various theories about what the chart depicts. Sure, you could go with the simple "I blew up!" But what does that actually mean? Did you run out of glycogen in your muscles? Probably not. Research on endurance athletes has found that when runners and cyclists hit the wall and pull the plug, due to seemingly insurmountable fatigue, they still have ample amounts of glycogen in their muscle stores and untapped muscle fibers at their disposal. Were you too loaded up on lactate? Maybe, especially if you gunned it from the start and started sucking wind 4 minutes later. In that case, you've flooded the system with lactate faster than your body can use it for aerobic metabolism, and it's wreaking havoc on your muscles' ability to contract. But research finds that absolute lactate levels are a pretty poor

THE FREAK-OUT FLOWCHART

THE CLIMB	YOUR RELATIVE CALM
You roll onto the foot of the climb, puffy clouds dotting the bluebird skies in the distance.	Chill and effervescent as strawberry champagne on ice, cuz that's how you like it.
The road weaves around a bend, where it greets you with a 13-percent switchback . . .	Ha! I've totally got this. A little huffing and puffing makes you feel alive!
. . . followed by an 18-percent kicker . . .	Who dumped acid in my capillaries? Okay, stay calm. It can't get any steeper, and I'm sure it's not *that* much farther to the top.
. . . followed by an 8-percent stretch that seemingly wraps halfway around the world to Japan (unless you're actually in Japan) . . .	Ouf. Did I eat enough before this ride?
. . . followed by what is unmistakably another steeply pitched S-turn into the unknown.	Oh, look, isn't that swell? MORE EFFING SWITCHBACKS!! Are you *kidding* me? Seriously!? I mean, *seriously*. Maybe I should downsh . . . . Oh great! Out of gears. That's dandy. Wish I'd stashed a nice bottle of Chianti in my jersey to go with my roasted legs!
It seems to be leveling off . . .	Okay. You got this. Toss it in a bigger gear, get up, and ice this climb like a Manhattan cupcake.
. . . um, no . . . *not* leveling off	[Click . . . click . . . click . . . .] *Groan*. Wish I'd packed lights, because mine have just gone out . . . .

predictor of fatigue. So, while dwindling fuel and increasingly taxed muscles certainly can contribute to your implosion, evidence increasingly points elsewhere.

What's really happening has far less to do with your legs than you might think. A growing body of research reveals that fatigue comes less from your muscles than it does from your mind. And, sometimes, your mind will make you tired when your muscles could continue. Once you understand this continuous feedback loop, you can manipulate it to climb into the clouds . . . or at least get up that last big hill of the day.

CAPTAIN KIRK AND MR. SPOCK AT THE HELM

Think of your bike as *Star Trek's USS Enterprise*. Commanding it up Milky Way Lane are Captain James T. Kirk and his trusty sidekick Commander Spock, who represent parts of your brain.

Spock is all Mr. Conservative Logic. He's reading the dashboard, scanning the horizon, and calling the shots, based on potential outcomes calculated using reasoned permutations. He's keeping a constant, watchful eye on all of your metabolic metrics: the amount of fuel (glycogen) in your muscles and liver (which, remember, feeds both your legs and your brain); your core body temperature; your blood plasma levels (to help you sweat and cool down said core body temperature); the amount of damage your muscle fibers are withstanding, and so forth. If any one of those metabolic metrics starts looking bad, Spock will cut the engine and change course to protect you from harm.

On the other side sits the emotional, passionate, reward-seeking, and sometimes impetuous Captain Kirk. He's probably the one that got you on this hill in the first place. He wants you to succeed, maybe at all costs, but if things aren't looking good or he finds something better to do that will be more rewarding and less painful (like coasting down the mountain and finding an attractive alien to hang out with), he's wont to do that as well.

To climb your best, you need to keep both of these commanders happy and satisfied. That means using the same well-rounded training approach to condition your mind as you do to condition your muscles.

TRAINING SPOCK

Remember, Spock only wants to protect you. So, anything you can do to assuage his worried, logical mind will convince him to give you the green light to carry on when the hill gets hard. Here's what works.

KNOW THE PROFILE. Guys like Spock do not like surprises. They also don't like unknowns. They really hate surprising unknowns. So, when you round the bend of what you're *sure* must be the top of a long, hard climb, and you spy nothing but more tilted earth, he's going to start shutting you down. On the flip side, if you have done a little research on your route and you know the general duration and pitch of the climb, your Spock brain knows the anticipated end point and will be less apprehensive about your ability to complete the climb. If you have any doubts about the power of knowing the profile, consider the sprint finish phenomenon. You can be 100-percent cracked and basically crawling along, but the moment you spy the finish line, you suddenly have the energy to toss the hammer down and finish fast. Spock knows that you'll be done soon, so he gives all systems a go.

BANG OUT SOME INTERVALS. Intervals improve your climbing on myriad levels—most of which you read about in the previous chapters. One overlooked benefit is the mental one. Every time you put out a damn-the-torpedoes, full-throttle, all-out, holy-crap-that-hurts effort, you're teaching Spock that you can push past comfortable limits and still be okay.

As you get fitter and stronger, interval training also raises the warning point for all those metrics that Spock is monitoring—you burn more fat and spare precious glucose; you use lactate more effectively; your thermoregulation system is more finely tuned, so you're also able to move up the hill more quickly before Spock starts seeing warning signs.

TRY FASTED TRAINING. Fasted training—doing a couple easy rides on an empty stomach, like before breakfast—improves your metabolic flexibility, which will allow your Spock brain to stay chill when your glycogen is running low. In one study, researchers had a group of 20 cyclists follow the same diet and training regimen of 60- to 90-minute training rides each day. Half the group did their rides before breakfast. The other half ate their breakfasts about an hour-and-a-half beforehand. After 6 weeks, both groups improved their performance in a 60-minute time trial. However, the fasted group had significantly increased their levels of fat-burning enzymes and were better fat burners at all intensities than those who ate first. That means two things: One, the fasters were better able to spare their limited glycogen stores, so they could go longer without hitting the wall. Two, should they find themselves on a long climb with dipping glycogen levels, their Spock brain will be less likely to hit the panic button, because there's always plenty of fat to

⊚ FOOLING YOURSELF

One of the most compelling bits of evidence that you can indeed manipulate your highly analytical Spock brain to your advantage is the swish-and-spit studies that have been stacking up for the past decade. They've found that, when cyclists swish a carbohydrate sports drink in their mouths for 5 to 10 seconds and spit it out, they perform better (by about 2 percent) during 60-minute time trial tests and the exercise feels easier, compared to actually drinking the sports drink or swishing and spitting out an artificially sweetened placebo beverage. MRI studies find that regions of your brain light up just by the presence of carbs in your mouth. Sensing that fuel is on the way, the brain revs your engine and lets you go harder.

---

spare. Bonus: because your brain relies solely on glucose, being able to preserve it while burning fat will help to ensure that Spock (and Kirk) don't shut you down simply because they're starving. You don't need to do this every day to reap the benefits. Once or twice a week will do the trick.

STAY FUELED AND HYDRATED. This is a no-brainer, but one we all botch at one time or another. If your Spock brain is monitoring your well-being, maintain your mojo up those climbs by maintaining your nutrition and hydration (See "What to Eat While You Climb" on page 112 for more specifics). Also, be sure to start your hard hilly rides with your tank on full. Research on cyclists has found that your brain uses available fuel as one of the factors to set your pace for your ride. In one study, researchers found cyclists set their 60-minute time trial intensity within 2 minutes of starting, and that intensity was proportionate to the amount of glycogen they had stored going into the effort.

TRAINING KIRK

Henry Ford famously said, "Whether you think you can, or you think you can't—you're right." That should be hanging inspirational poster–style inside your emotional Captain Kirk brain, because the messages you give yourself when the going gets hard—like when you're 5,000 feet up Mount Lemmon in Tucson—hugely impact the ultimate outcome. Here's how to train your Kirk brain to conquer any climb.

BE YOUR OWN CHEERLEADER. Remember in the 2017 Super Bowl, when the Patriots were down against the Falcons 28 to 3 in the third quarter, and everyone packed up their chips and guac and called it a night . . . only to awaken to the news that the New England powerhouse had racked up 25 unanswered points in the fourth quarter and another 6 to win the thing in overtime? You think Patriots coach Bill Belichick went into the locker room at halftime and said, "You losers suck! You'll never beat these guys! Might as well take up golf." No. And you shouldn't talk to yourself like that either, no matter how slow and pained you feel up any given climb.

Negative self-talk changes your brain chemistry and becomes a self-fulfilling prophecy. Positive self-talk has the opposite effect. When scientists pored through 32 sports psychology studies, they found that motivational self-talk like "I am strong. I can do this." can significantly improve endurance performance. In another cycling study, scientists had 24 athletes hammer out a time trial (TT) to exhaustion. Then, half the group was instructed to develop four motivational statements—two for the early part of the TT, and two for the later stages—to practice during their rides. When all the cyclists came back for retesting 2 weeks later, the positive self-talkers improved by 18 percent! The control group saw no improvement.

Pro tip: Amp up the positive self-talk benefits by addressing yourself by name and you rather than I,—"Okay, Sam, you've got this. You're feeling steady and strong."—a trick that is popular among pro athletes. Research finds that this subtle linguistic shift tricks your brain into treating you like another person—and many of us are kinder to others than we are to ourselves.

TUNE IN, TUNE OUT, SING A TUNE. Say you're trying to set a personal best on a hilly Gran Fondo or long hill climb. Do you funnel your focus into your breathing, pedal stroke mechanics, and muscle sensations? Or, do you turn your focus outward on the scenery, start working math problems in your head, or mentally sing a tune? Exercise scientists have long debated the benefits of associating (the former) with dissociating (the latter) on exercise performance. As you might imagine, they both serve a purpose, and the best athletes have the ability to switch back and forth between the two, as needed.

In the case of a long climb or hilly event, it helps to associate more in the beginning. Are you pacing yourself properly? Have you placed yourself in a good position in the pack? Are you pushing the right gear? At what point will you need food and fluids? Those thoughts make your Spock brain happy and keep the Kirk side distracted. As you pedal farther into the challenge and things start to get uncomfortable, honing in on that discomfort can become counterproductive, as your Kirk brain starts questioning the wisdom in all this. That's when pivoting your attention outward comes into play. Instead of cuing in on how badly your legs are burning up the crest of a steep climb, count pedal strokes to the next mailbox or count backward from 10, over and over, until you reach the top. At mile 78 of a 100-miler, when everything is starting to ache, play the alphabet game working from A to Z of places in the world you'd like to visit, or put a favorite song in your head and sing every verse to yourself as you pedal to the rhythm. Switching back and forth between the two approaches will help keep you on task—maintaining a proper cadence and pace and staying on top of your nutrition and hydration—while also giving you a much-needed mental break when fatigue sets in.

USE YOUR BREATH. There's a reason that people say, "Take a deep breath." when someone is freaking out. The act of taking a full, deep breath stimulates the parasympathetic system, prompting you to calm down and sharpen your focus. Huffing and puffing has the opposite effect and is controlled by your sympathetic nervous system as part of the fight-or-flight response, that stress hormone–fueled state that is anything but calm. There's room for both when you're charging up a climb—especially if you're gunning for a personal best. But, controlled breathing is best to keep your Kirk brain collected when you're working your way up a long, steep climb—and that means breathing into your belly to fully expand your diaphragm rather than relying on less-efficient, less-effective shallow chest breathing.

To do it, pull your breath deep into your torso until your abdomen expands. Then, exhale completely and repeat. This type of full belly breathing not only ensures that you're tapping into your full lung capacity and using as many alveoli (the grape-shaped air sacs that line your lungs) as possible, which is vital for maximum oxygen exchange, but also serves the dual purpose of keeping you calm and in control.

Pro tip: When the going gets hard, synchronize your breathing to your pedal stroke. To do it, fall into a cadence where you're exhaling at the top of your pedal strokes and inhaling around the upstroke, alternating legs, pushing out your air to the rhythm of your effort. For moderate climbs, breathe in for three counts and out for two counts. On particularly long, steep hills, shift to a three-count pattern, breathing in for two and out forcefully for one.

I culled this technique from Budd Coates, an Olympic trials marathoner, exercise physiologist, and co-author of *Runner's World Running on Air,* and ran it by respiratory researcher Paul W. Davenport, PhD, of the University of Florida. Dr. Davenport confirmed that synchronized breathing can boost performance by ensuring that you're taking even, complete breaths and using the force of your exhalations to push your pedals, much like a weightlifter uses the exhale to hoist a heavy barbell. It never lets me down while I'm working my way up.

FEED YOUR HEAD

Your brain lives on glucose (sugar) alone. It burns 6 to 7 grams of sugar (the amount in two Hershey's Kisses) each hour just to keep you living and breathing. Once you start jamming up an 11-percent grade? Better fire up the chocolate factory. When brain glucose runs low, your levels of adenosine and serotonin rise, which causes fatigue, and your levels of dopamine drop, which interferes with your concentration and makes way for negative thoughts to bubble up. Mental fatigue can weaken muscle contractions up to 25 percent. When I'm on a long climb and the demon voices start piping up telling me that I'm just not strong enough or good enough, more often than not, popping an energy chew will silence them and make me feel nearly instantly better.

THE ART OF DANCING UP THE MOUNTAINS

You can be a walking pair of lungs atop a set of monster quads and still struggle up climbs without the right pacing, approach, and technique. Maestros of the mountains ascend with such grace and ease by employing all these mental strategies along with smart technique. Here's how to pull it all together.

TOP OFF AT THE BOTTOM. If it's been a while since you've eaten and/or if you're heading into a particularly long climb, give yourself a shot of fuel at the base of the climb, before you start. You'll get a nice energy boost, and it's far easier to take a bite of a banana or bar when you're rolling easy on the relative flats than once you're borderline hypoxic and seeing spots on the climb.

THINK LIGHT; RIDE QUIET. Apply what fellow coach and climbing specialist Andy Applegate calls Qigong climbing, a technique that blends positive thinking with relaxed technique. As you approach the climb, think "light" thoughts—clouds, birds, angels, whatever lightens up your mental space. Then, start with your face and progressively relax your body down to your feet, being sure to release any unnecessary tension, particularly in your shoulders, which should be down and relaxed, and your hands, which should be loosely gripping the bars (not white-knuckling them). "You want your upper body so quiet that if someone were to film you from the waist up, they wouldn't be able to tell if you were climbing or just riding along," Applegate says.

Apply the same quiet posture approach when you stand. Keep your shoulders squared and facing forward, as if you were balancing beer glasses on them. Avoid dropping them from side to side, which will waste energy and send you weaving up the slope like a drunken paperboy.

MAINTAIN YOUR POWER POSITION. Remember, that full breath thing is important. Facilitate that by keeping your back straight and chest open to allow maximum airflow into your lungs. Relax your arms so that your elbows are outside of your hips. When it's time to stand, click into the next bigger gear, and stand on the top of the pedal stroke to minimize loss of momentum. Stand

(continued on page 86)

WISDOM FROM THE MOUNTAINSIDE

There are many ways up the mountain, but coaches and athletes pull out these mental tricks for a little psychic push.

"Riders often feel isolated and in their own heads up a long climb. They'll think, 'I have 4 more miles. How can I possibly do this for 4 more miles?!' Don't even think about that. Breathe in and breathe out, counting your breaths to quiet your mind. Then, keep your mind in the moment. What do you see around you? Check out the views. Note all the little things along the way. You can always keep pedaling in that moment. It's only when you look too far ahead that you start to shut yourself down. The hill won't last forever, but the rewards of reaching the top will. That confidence transcends cycling, as does the ability to simply focus on the task at hand at any given moment, rather than being buried by the larger job you're trying to accomplish."
—**Ian Marling, 30, coach with Bell Lap Coaching in Massachusetts**

"People talk about suffering on the bike. I work with juveniles in the criminal justice system who have violent pasts and lives and have seen murders before age 12 and have suffered far more than most of us will ever imagine. When I think about bicycling, no matter how hard I'm pushing myself, that's not really suffering. Mount Washington is a speed

bump compared to that. Stay in the moment, and keep your perspective. It's just a climb."
—**Jonathan Simmons, 56, former Peaks Coaching Group athlete from Cape Cod, Massachusetts**

"Being uncomfortable is not the end of the world. Even those riders at the front of the climb are uncomfortable. Everyone is! To be a successful climber, you have to be comfortable being uncomfortable for a while."
—**Victoria Di Savino, 38, of Buffalo, hill climb specialist and Mount Washington Hillclimb winner**

"Rather than trying to conquer the whole climb at once, I will often set little goals along the way. Use a landmark like a utility pole or a mailbox, if this is a regular route, and try to stay in the saddle until reaching that point, only standing once past that point. On really difficult and particularly long climbs, I do repeated counts to 10 say to the next corner or some other point. On 'deadly climbs,' I will do this over and over again. It's just a mind game, but it seems to work for me."
—**Sherman Cravens, 60, Peaks Coaching Athlete in Bedford, Virginia**

"The longer the hill, the greater the ability for dissociative thinking. Bury and lose yourself in the grind, and keep your pedals turning."
—**Mark Graves, 56, recreational rider in Stratford, Ontario, who recently took a summer to pedal from his home all the way to Leadville, Colorado, to finish his fourth Leadville 100 mountain bike race**

with your rear end over the saddle, keeping your weight centered over the bottom bracket. Avoid leaning forward, which unweights the rear and can cause skidding, or make you inadvertently toss your bike backward, which is alarming and potentially dangerous for any riders who may be close behind. You should feel like you're running (albeit slowly and deliberately) on the pedals, allowing the bike to rock gently, but not excessively, from side to side.

GIVE YOUR LEGS A HELPING HAND. When the grade gets so steep that you're sliding into standstill (and topple) territory, tuck your elbows into your sides, dip your torso toward the bars, and gently but firmly pull back on the bars with every downstroke. This lets you transfer power from your upper body through your core and into your legs to assist you in forward progress.

FINISH FASTER THAN YOU BEGIN. You don't beat a giant by going after its feet; you take aim at the head. Remember that as you ride up your next monster climb. Rather than attacking the foot of the climb and petering out before you reach the summit, dial back your pace until it feels easier than you want it to, just below your lactate threshold or FTP. Then, ramp up your speed as you get closer to the top, and attack over the summit—and likely sail by everyone who is collapsing from starting out too fast.

CHANNEL YOUR MOJO. No matter how many butterflies you visualize and happy songs you put into your head and how well you eat and drink, you're bound to have spells of sinking morale on long, hard, hilly days, especially if you're doing consecutive long, hard, hilly days in a bike tour or multiday ride. That's when some visual aids help. During the Pennsylvania Perimeter Ride Against Cancer (PPRAC), a hellishly hilly 7-day ride I do every 2 years, riders tape pictures of loved ones who have battled (and maybe lost the battle to) cancer to their top tubes for inspiration. Even pro riders will tape photos and inspiring messages to their bikes for added inspiration. As professional cyclocross rider Jeremy Powers once told *Bicycling* magazine, when all else fails, "this will give you something to focus on besides the pain in your legs and lungs."

So, now, let's go back to "The Freak-Out Flowchart" from page 76 and make it right.

CLIMBING ZEN FLOWCHART

THE CLIMB	YOUR RELATIVE CALM
You roll onto the foot of the climb, puffy clouds dotting the bluebird skies in the distance.	Chill and effervescent as strawberry champagne on ice, cuz that's how you like it . . . . Just remember to pop a little fuel in your gullet to keep your mind and muscles as happy later as they are now.
The road weaves around a bend, where it greets you with a 13-percent switchback . . .	I'd love to charge and attack, but it's time to settle in and keep the effort below threshold to save those matches.
. . . followed by an 18-percent kicker . . .	Little click of the gearing and out of the saddle. Nice and smooth, gently rocking the bike and beelining it up the grade.
. . . followed by an 8-percent stretch that seemingly wraps halfway around the world to Japan (unless you're actually in Japan) . . .	1-2-3, 1-2-3—breathe in and out, pressing pedals in sync with my inhalations and exhalations . . . smooth and strong and steady.
. . . followed by what is unmistakably another steeply pitched S-turn into the unknown.	Okay. You've got this. It's just a hill. You're strong. You're steady. You've got this . . . .
It seems to be leveling off . . .	Deep breaths. Take a hit off your bottle to keep cool and hydrated. Spin out your legs for a micro-recovery, just in case this really isn't the end.
. . . um, no . . . *not* leveling off	Good thing I got that drink. Brace that core, pull gently on the bars, keep counting and thinking positive thoughts. You got this.

F%CK! | **87**

7 | WHEELS IN THE SKY

Sometimes it is about the bike: the right gear—and gearing—can transform mountains into molehills.

▶ **NOT BEING ONE TO** overthink things (or, honestly, sometimes adequately think things), I never really gave much thought to my gears during many of my years of riding and competing. Whatever was on the bike I was riding was what I was training and racing with. Fussing with gears and cassettes and the like just seemed like more work than it was worth. Then came Mount Washington—the infamous race up arguably one of the toughest climbs on the planet.

During the weeks leading up to it, I started getting a little panicky as I watched my husband, Dave, diligently studying the mountain's gradients and preparing his bike, swapping his road setup for a compact crankset and searching for places to shave weight. I hadn't thought twice about my bike.

So, I asked my friend Bill, who'd done it twice. "Do I need a compact?" We rambled back and forth about the event and its demands, ultimately deciding that I'd be fine with my 53/39T. I was at peace with that decision until Dave,

Brian (our friend and chauffeur for the day), and I pulled up to the venue. I looked at the start, which was easily a 12-percent grade. My jaw agape, I looked at Brian. He smiled and said, "It's pretty much that way all the way to the top, until it turns to 22 percent."

"I am a complete idiot," I thought. So went my train of thought for about the first 3 miles.

The event starts at the base of the mountain. They fire a cannon, and off you go for about 100 yards before you bang a left and are immediately greeted with a 12.5-percent grade. The mountain then undulates between about 10 and 18 percent for 7.5 miles, until the very top, when it does indeed ratchet up to 22 percent for the final 50 yards. I was in a good position as we rounded the bend and started climbing, but within 30 seconds, I'd already dropped into my lowest gear and was muscling my way through pretty much every pedal stroke.

"This isn't good," I thought, looking up and seeing nothing but a relentless pitch ahead. "Why didn't you switch your gears? Can you do this for more than 7 miles? This is supposed to be the 'easy' part . . . " I kept my head down and kept grinding.

Meanwhile, already pretty far up the hill ahead of me was Marti Shea, comfortably (or as comfortable as one can be on that hill!) spinning her compact chainring and 11-32 cassette (more on all those numbers in a bit). She would go on to win that day . . . and bag 11 total Mount Washington titles before hanging up her racing wheels in 2015.

Myself? As noted earlier, I self-talked, willed, and worked my way up to a third-place finish. But, it wasn't pretty, and I'm pretty certain I wouldn't be able to repeat the performance without toppling over like the last wobbling pin in a perfect strike.

I felt a wee bit better when I read an article Shea penned for *Bicycling* magazine a few years after that fateful day, in which she confessed to making the same blunder early on. "In my opinion, most people are overgeared for climbing—equating tiny cogs and big rings with being tougher and stronger," she said. "When I first started climbing Mount Washington . . . I used traditional gearing. The only way for me to get up the mountain was to stand almost the entire way, and pedal with an average cadence of 55. I did that for about 4 years and won with it. But, I realized I wasn't getting any faster!"

So, she started experimenting. "I switched to a compact up front 50/34 with a regular 11–28 cassette in rear, and I went a little faster. Then, the next year, I ran a compact up front with an 11–32 in rear. I went faster again. Then, the next year, I went 11–36 in rear, and I ran that for a few years. Finally, in 2012, I did all-out mountain bike gearing! I ran a 22 up front with an 11–28 in rear, and that was the fastest I ever rode. So, I got older, but I got faster! I went back to regular gearing at age 43 and did 69 minutes. Finally, at the ripe old age of 49, I did 63 minutes running the 22 upfront with the 11–28 in rear."

The magic was in the cadence, she says. "I found that I could sit and spin a high cadence. Gone were the heavy legs and the lactic acid accumulation."

She's not alone in her hard-won wisdom. While it may feel pretty badass to conquer a massive climb in a monster gear, long gone are the days of pushing tall, heavy gears uphill. Even World Tour riders now use big cassettes that would have marked them as a "Fred" (a derogatory term for a clueless, uncool cyclist) just 5 or 10 years ago. So, if you haven't given even so much as a passing thought to your gears (and some of your gear), now's the time.

By adjusting your gears to the terrain you want to tackle, you can stay far fresher and avoid injury, as you make your way over even the most relentless mountain rides. While we're talking gears and gear, there are some weight-saving swaps and smart bike setup hacks that can give you a leg up when you're out trying to crush it on the climbs.

GEAR RATIOS AND RATIONALES

Starting with the very basics: Let's look at the drivetrain, which consists of your cranks and chainrings, which are mounted to your bike's bottom bracket, as well as your cassette (sometimes also called a cluster or freewheel), which is mounted to the hub of the rear wheel. The chainrings and cassette are connected by the chain. It's the combination of chainrings and cogs on the cassette that creates what we know as our gears.

Depending on your setup, there will be anywhere from a single chainring to three chainrings in the front. On the rear wheel, your cassette will be outfitted with 8 to 12 cogs. The combination of the two produces what's known as gear development—the distance your bike travels in one revolution of the crankset. High gears propel the bike farther per revolution. Lower ones propel it shorter distances. That's the easy part. The harder part is configuring the sweet spot of gearing that allows you to climb at a healthy cadence—e.g., not lower than 60 rpm, even when the going gets tough—while still giving you high enough gears that you're not spun out (at a place where you can't go any faster because your pedaling rpm is maxed out and there are no high gears left).

Let's look at the chainrings first. Traditional road gearing (which incidentally is becoming less traditional with every passing year) is typically a double chainring configuration with a 53-tooth outer chainring and a 39-tooth inner chainring. That's a pretty stout combination but well-suited for flat to rolling roads. Once you start turning cranks on more vertical terrain, however, you may find yourself searching for that one more gear that isn't there, which is not only demoralizing but hard on your back and knees, as you are forced to torque your way to the top.

That's why many manufacturers are offering—and many riders are opting for—bikes outfitted with a 52/36T chainring combo (known as semi- or mid-compact gearing) or even a 50/34T pairing (known as compact gearing). The smaller chainrings simply offer greater opportunity for spinning a higher cadence, even up the steepest terrain.

The next choice is cassette. Keeping in mind that small cogs are "higher" gears and large cogs are "lower" gears, you can choose among a variety of configurations. On the road side, you'll commonly find cassettes with 10 or 11 cogs ranging from 11-tooth or 12-tooth up to 28-tooth or even 32-tooth, for extreme conditions.

To maximize the effectiveness of the chainring configuration you select in the front, you need to pair it with the most complementary cog range in the rear. The goal here is to give yourself the widest usable gear range for your type of riding. If you run a compact crank in the front, try pairing it with a wider-range cassette on the back, such as an 11–28 versus a 12–26. That way you end up with nearly as many gear inches out of your downhill gear as you would with a traditional crankset, but you have far more flexibility for climbing hills.

🔷 TRIPLE THREAT?

Years ago, it was common for road bikes to come with three front chainrings, known as triples, where there was an inner 30T ring added to the double 52/39T crankset (mountain bikes usually came stock with 22/32/44T combinations). Road triples were especially common on touring bikes, since if you're traveling across a state or country, you're going to want *all* the gears. Nowadays, however, triples are starting to fade into the history books, as compacts and wide-range cassettes fill most gearing needs without the extra weight, duplicate gears, and cumbersome shifting that come along with that extra ring.

On the mountain bike side, front chainrings are often smaller than on the road side. Companies aim to make mountain bikes lighter and less prone to mechanical mishaps (which are far more common when you're cranking through streams, hopping logs, and negotiating rugged terrain that may be muddy, sandy, dusty, or all of the above). Many bikes are now coming stocked with a single front 30T or 32T ring, though you can go as low as 26T or as high as 40T.

To accommodate this shift to 1x gearing, mountain bike cassettes have ventured into *extreme* territory, with some bikes now coming outfitted with ginormous 10–50 (yes, five-0) cassettes, which makes the biggest cog on the back of those mountain bikes as big as the big ring on a compact-crank road bike. (And truly with a 30–50 as your low gear, you should be able to scale walls like Spiderman).

When opting for a 1x setup, the thing to remember is that your gear selection is broad, but still somewhat limited. Even if you have an 11-cog cassette, that's still 11 gears, as opposed to 20 gears at your disposal with a more classic two-chainring drivetrain. If you ride Leadville-style events, where you're spending long hours pedaling over extreme variations in terrain, sticking with more conventional 2x gearing, where you can choose a 22T or 24T small ring and 36T or 38T large ring paired to a 11–36 cassette, may be the wiser choice, as it can help you maintain an optimal cadence and power output throughout the entire ride.

WHERE THE RUBBER MEETS THE ROAD

You have enough trouble contending with Earth's gravitational pull when you're climbing, so the last thing you want is unnecessary resistance from the road. For years—heck decades—we thought that meant buying the skinniest tires you could tolerate. For most racers and riders, 23mm pumped to a rock hard 100+ psi was the norm, with some even opting for 19mms, which are like the Virginia Slims of racing rubber, in hopes of having the fastest-rolling, most-aerodynamic, least-resistant tire setup possible.

Well, it was all wrong. Not only are brick-solid skinny tires ungodly uncomfortable, as your body absorbs every stutter bump in the road, but also research shows that, pound for pound of psi, they have *more* rolling resistance. Isn't it ironic? Don't you think? Having Ping-Ponged my way up and down many a rough mountain road in the good old days, yes, I really do think it's ironic. But, it's also 100 percent scientific: At the same air pressure, 25mm tires actually experience less rolling resistance than their skinnier counterparts.

It's all about what scientists who study these things call the contact patch, which, as it sounds, is how much of your tire makes contact with the ground surface. On a narrow tire, the tire deforms or flattens along its length as you ride, so the contact patch is narrow but long on the pavement. A wider tire spreads out across its width, so you have a wider but shorter contact patch. The wider tire ultimately maintains a rounder shape, and rounder shapes roll faster.

Of course, when going wider, you have to consider weight, and you don't want to be dragging wagon wheels up an Alpine climb. But, the increased comfort and stability without the expense of increased resistance have made 25mms pretty much standard these days. Even in the pro peloton, if you take a look at the hoops on the start line, the majority are dressed with 25mm tires. In the Classics (one-day European pro-cycling races typically held in the spring) and on many Gran Fondos (timed amateur events) where riders traverse cobbles, B-roads, and plenty of rough terrain, you'll see 28s and above, especially now that so many bikes come with disc brakes, which leave loads of clearance between even a fat tire and the frame.

Wider tires also decrease your risk for getting a pinch flat while you're sailing down the other side of the climb because you have more real estate for the tire to compress before the rim hits the rubber and causes a snakebite (a pinch flat on both sides of the tube). One word of caution: The width of the tire and the width of the rim should correlate fairly closely. It makes the whole setup more aerodynamic, which also helps to lower the total resistance you have to overcome.

When it comes to how much pressure to run, that takes some experimentation. Err on the lower end of the recommended range when riding on rough and/or wet roads. Err on the higher side for smooth, dry pavement.

On the mountain bike side, ground contact is everything. And, it's funny, even though fat tires have always been part of what makes mountain biking mountain biking, the tires are still trending wider, with 27.5+ sized tires coming in at 2.8 to 3 inches across. You can run these at ridiculously low pressure and still enjoy trail-biting, never-slip traction up the steepest of steeps. Again, more tire means more weight. So, you need to figure out how much your need for increased traction balances out with your need for a lighter bike.

The same is true for cyclocross or gravel bikes, of course. Tire width and pressure is largely dependent on surface conditions. When traction is elusive, wider and lower tends to be better. When the ground is firmer and easier to grip, you can go with less tire and a firmer setup to save weight.

SET UP FOR SUCCESS

Watch Grand Tour riders in the miles before a major climb, and you'll see them tossing water bottles, emptying pockets, maybe even peeing off the side of the bike—doing anything and everything they can to shave weight, so they're lighter when they start their ascent. Obviously, you're not going to litter the roadside

⬀ DRESS FOR SUCCESS

There are some lessons you learn the hard way—and there are some you just keep learning the hard way, hoping each time that you won't have to relearn said lesson. This has been the story of my life, with dressing for days of climbing in the mountains where the temperatures can swing from 70°F at the base to 50°F at the top, and the weather can change from bright and sunny to buckets dumping from the sky in the click of a shifter. In these conditions, it's nearly always easy enough to stay warm on your way up the mountain. The big challenge is keeping yourself from going hypothermic on the way down, especially since you can find yourself descending for the better part of an hour!

Once, after ascending Mount Baldy—a 13-mile climb outside Los Angeles that gains more than 2,000 feet in the final 4.5 miles, topping out at an elevation of about 6,500 feet—I was dripping with sweat... and then, it started to snow. I was shuddering so terribly on the descent, I couldn't work my brakes and my bike was weaving underneath my unsteady legs. I had to pull off the road and huddle behind the tailpipe of an idling bus to warm up enough to continue. Don't do that. Plan ahead and bring what you need for the conditions you may face.

As a general rule of thumb, plan on the temperature dropping between 3° and 5°F for every 1,000 feet of elevation you gain. Also count on wind—even if it's not windy—because, when you're sailing downhill at 20, 30, 40, or even 50 mph, you're going to be plunging through the air and creating your own wind-chill effect. With that in mind, wear and/or pack the following:

BASE LAYER: Keeping your core comfortable is priority number one, because when your core gets cold, your body constricts vessels at your extremities to protect it. That means everything else feels cold. A comfortable core starts with a light layer against your skin. The base layer's job

---

with your GU wrappers and empty bottles on your rides, but if climbing is your thing, it's well worth it to look at your bike with a critical eye, and make some smart substitutions that will save grams—and sometimes pounds—in the fight against gravity. Use these easy ways to lighten your load.

SWAP WHEELS. Your rotating weight—wheels, tires, tubes (if you have

is to pull moisture away from your skin and move it to your outer layers, where it can evaporate. This helps keep you cool in the summer and prevents you from getting damp and cold in the winter. You can find insulating and noninsulating base layers. As the name suggests, insulating layers are made of materials that trap the heat your body is generating, while wicking the moisture away. They're obviously the garment of choice for cool-weather outings.

MID-LAYER: When the temperatures are moderate to mild, this will be your jersey (and possibly arm warmers). If it's cold, this could be a second base layer, with another level of insulation. Some days, this might be all you need, but if you're heading into the big mountains, you should definitely pack outer layers in your pockets, even if you don't need to wear them when you start out.

WIND/WEATHER LAYER: Your outer layer or layers are key for climbing comfort. It's worth investing in a quality vest and a really good, packable wind- and water-repellent jacket that you can slip on and off as conditions and temperatures vary while you make your way up and down the mountains. Look for ones that are made of durable, breathable materials like Gore-Tex. You'll be glad you did.

ACCESSORIES: You'll want gloves to keep your hands protected from the elements. For long days, slipping a spare pair in your pocket can be a luxurious spirit-lifter, as you can pull on a fresh, dry pair when the ones you're wearing are soaked with sweat. I'm also a huge fan of what we Philadelphia cyclists call the neck jawn—or gaiter. Buff is the classic brand, but you can find them through various manufacturers in any number of materials. Your neck is a very vulnerable spot for chilly air and nearly impossible to keep warm when you're descending. A light wrap around your neck will prevent you from tensing up with your shoulders around your ears on long, brisk descents.

---

them), etc.—is what you feel most keenly when you climb, because it's what you must keep in motion with every single pedal stroke. That's just physics. Switching from aluminum to carbon fiber wheels can make you feel like you've sprouted wings. This is probably the single best upgrade you can make to significantly improve climbing performance.

⊙ STRAVA!

Quite obviously, you don't *need* to use Strava—a popular social fitness app that lets you track your performance and compare it with other users—to enjoy hill climbing. But Strava, which bestows you with virtual bling in the form of medals and King and Queen of the Mountain crowns for personal bests and top-level performances, can be extremely motivating.

Strava not only inspires you to keep improving but also it issues various challenges throughout the year. So, if you need a motivation boost, you can join a climbing challenge, where you earn a special Strava badge for climbing 8,000 meters (26,000+ feet) in a single month.

As Strava's popularity skyrockets into the stratosphere (users have recorded more than a billion activities and 100,000 new riders join every 40 days), this virtual reality is also starting to seep into the physical world. In County Clare, Ireland, county officials have actually installed signposts marking the start and finish of popular Strava climbing segments.

SWITCH TIRES. With the obvious caveat that lighter tires tend to be more susceptible to punctures, lighter race tires roll substantially faster. When I do fat bike races in the winter, I can save more than a full pound on my bike by switching to lighter tires. Switching to light latex tubes is also an easy way to shed a few grams.

DITCH THAT BULKY BAG. Still have a saddlebag swinging in the breeze behind you? Drop all that heavy canvas casing in favor of a lighter saddle strap, which will hold all your gear without the excess weight. You will still have everything you need, but without the bulky material you don't.

CLEAN YOUR BIKE. Unless you rally the thing through mud bogs, it's not likely weighed down with caked-on dirt, but a clean drivetrain runs more smoothly with less friction and resistance and that's free, easy speed.

8 | WEIGHTY MATTERS

Eating like a bird doesn't guarantee that you'll fly uphill, so here's how to eat on and off the bike for climbing success . . . and why you shouldn't get too hung up on weight.

▶ **BACK IN 2015,** I had the privilege to ride the entire length of the AMGEN Tour of California as part of Team GU's six-rider squad. We pedaled more than 560 miles and climbed more than 43,400 feet over the course of 7 days. To say that our intrepid little team of cyclists, including GU's CEO (chief endurance officer), Brian Vaughan, were fretting over our training, fitness, nutrition, and race weight would be just a slight understatement.

Our fret level turned to pure freak out when, the day before our big adventure, in the name of science and hydration tracking (and I think because he thought we'd all get Team Sky-level lean), Brian whipped out a few scales. He wanted us to weigh in before the journey started and before and after each stage. The first teammate climbed on. Eyes pop. Jaw drops. "That's not what my scale says at home!" He stepped off. Stepped on another scale . . . . then silently shook his head and jotted down the result on the communal clipboard. The next teammate climbed on. Severe frown.

More exclamations of incredulousness. More head shaking and number jotting. My turn: 134 pounds, which is about 4 pounds heavier than my usual weight.

And, so it continues. Now, we're all about to embark on this behemoth week wigging out about being weighted down. And, it only got worse. By Saturday—the Queen Stage that ends on the summit of the notorious Mount Baldy (see page 145)—we were all pushing maximum density. When I placed my feet on the smooth, cool, plastic surface I'd grown to loathe, I was more than 137 pounds. Another teammate stepped on next, looked at me, and said, "My body is totally f****d up!" I laughed and assured him that we'd be fine. . . . And, we were.

Morning scale freak-outs aside, we crushed it, finishing strong and fast every day through wild spring conditions that ranged from blazing heat to cold sheets of rain. Despite starting 4 pounds heavier than my ideal climbing weight (based on popular formulas), I collected 19 Strava QOMs over the course of the tour. On Baldy day (staring down 86 miles and more than 12,000 feet of climbing), when I tipped the scales 7 pounds over fighting weight, I punched my way up the Strava leaderboard to second overall on the 8-mile stretch from Firehouse to Village on Baldy Road, as well as on the steepest segments of Baldy Charge (11 percent) and the nearly mile-long Bowling Alley stretch that averages 10 percent.

WHAT IS "WEIGHT" ANYWAY?

Once back on home turf, I went on to have some of my best race performances at 134 to 135 pounds—and some of my worst days at what should have been my "best" weight, several pounds lighter. The takeaway for me, over the years: Making weight a goal can be a losing proposition. Being well-fueled and -hydrated with fully stocked stores is more important than any number on a scale. Oh, and there are also many ways to gain weight; some more productive than others.

To illustrate the point, I'll share a little experiment I started a few years back, which has become a permanent habit. While running various weight-loss plans for magazine features and personal clients, I've long wrestled with advising how often people should or should not weigh themselves. On one hand, the evidence is nearly unequivocal that people who step on the scale regularly, at least once a week, if not daily, are not only more likely to be successful in their weight-loss efforts but also are more likely to keep their weight down (the toughest part for most folks). The downside is that it's easy—especially for hardworking overachievers—to develop an unhealthy obsession with the numbers on the scale.

For that latter reason, I had personally stayed away from scales for most of my adult life. I preferred to just go by feel—by how my clothes fit, by how I felt on the bike, by how I felt about the image in the mirror. But, I had to be honest with myself. That never really worked perfectly. I ended up feeling out of touch with my physical self. So, then, I started weighing myself just once every few weeks or so, always with a bit of trepidation—just to check in. That worked okay. At least I could see when my weight was drifting up and down. These occasional weigh-ins gave me a bit more control over my weight, but my understanding of what influenced it was still lacking.

I knew the basics, of course. Eat too much, move too little, you gain weight. Eat less, move more, you lose weight. Eat just right, move just right, you maintain. Or, at least that's what we in the fitness industry like to tell people, because it's a tidy answer. I'd long had the sneaking suspicion that it's a bit of bull, however. While running numerous diet-and-exercise test panels for various magazines, I'd see firsthand how some folks dropped multiple pounds seemingly overnight, while others could barely make the numbers budge, no matter how diligently they stuck to the plan. I confess that, often, I just figured the "nonresponders" weren't really following the plan. I mean, if they were, why weren't they losing weight? (As an aside, I'd like to apologize to those people. And to that one particular client I had a few years back who insisted—to my insistent denial that it was possible—that he would gain 4 pounds overnight. I'm really sorry. You were right. I was wrong.)

So, I decided that I would weigh myself each and every morning that I was home (I didn't take the scale on bike trips), and see how my weight tracked according to my training and what was going on in my life. It was extremely eye-opening.

I'll start out with this: You have likely read (and I have written) that one pound equals 3,500 calories. To lose a pound a week, traditional wisdom says that you need to cut back or burn off an additional 500 calories a day. Logic follows that to put on a pound a week, you need to increase your intake by the same 500 calories. Well, all that works on paper. But, we humans are not the products of origami, and true weight gain and loss is as complicated, if not more, than making a human being out of folding paper. The number you see on the scale is obviously not just fat. It's muscle and bone and water, and everything else you're made of. Weight gain and loss involves all of it, and it's not such a neat equation.

Case in point: Here's a snippet from a summer when I was racing and riding lots. Check out the bolded numbers below. The week in between it looks like I must've gone on a pizza-and-pastry binge. Instead, I had just come off of an arduous 6-day charity ride that covered 560 miles and 33,000 feet of climbing. I came home feeling like my legs were water balloons, and the scale reflected that—a 5-pound gain. And, no, I hadn't taken in an additional 17,500 calories to gain 5 pounds.

7/26/13, 6:40 a.m. 133.0 lbs.
7/27/13, 7:25 a.m. 132.2 lbs.
8/4/13, 9:25 a.m. 137.0 lbs.
8/5/13, 7:01 a.m. 135.2 lbs.
8/6/13, 7:05 a.m. 132.6 lbs.
8/7/13, 6:54 a.m. 134.4 lbs.
8/8/13, 6:24 a.m. 132.6 lbs.
8/9/13, 6:57 a.m. 131.6 lbs.

My go-to physiology expert, Stacy Sims, PhD, senior research fellow at the Adams High Performance Centre at the University of Waikato in New Zealand, assured me that all the effort had just put my body in super-compensation mode—i.e., my body had increased its plasma volume and stuffed my glycogen stores to the gills with carbs and water, preparing for another 100 miles on the road. Hard efforts also create inflammation in the muscles—i.e., more fluid gain. The poundage I had put on was truly mostly "water weight." When I was back to my normal routine, my body let it go, and the pounds came off.

Here's another week a little later on during the same calendar year.

12/4/13, 6:38 a.m. 130.8 lbs.
12/5/13, 6:38 a.m. 131.2 lbs.
12/6/13, 6:24 a.m. 130.0 lbs.
12/9/13, 9:20 a.m. 137.2 lbs.
12/10/13, 7:33 a.m. 135.4 lbs.
12/11/13, 6:26 a.m. 133.2 lbs.
12/12/13, 6:34 a.m. 131.4 lbs.

What happened here was a case study in the opposite of healthy direction. It was single-speed cyclocross world championships weekend in Philly. A group of us were flopping in an unfurnished apartment with nothing in the cupboards but doughnut holes and whiskey. Sleep was nonexistent, as was breakfast. I think I managed one healthy meal. Though I ate very little, it was generally something awful and usually around 11:00 p.m. On top of that, we were spending hours riding and racing our single-speed bikes, leading to very loaded up (literally) legs. The numbers speak for themselves. My body, perhaps sensing the apocalypse was upon us, had gone into full-on survival mode, hanging on to whatever it could, leaving me bloated like a dog tick. Again, after a few days of normalcy, I settled back to where I belong.

I've learned other things, too. Like a big night at the sushi bar leaves me bloated the next day (soy sauce = water retention). When I eat according to hunger, I am shockingly weight-stable. When I don't, I drift, but that's okay because I know how to normalize. I taper really well (when I cut back on riding before a big event, I can store *lots* of carbs and water quickly). And, I blow through those stores well, too.

It was reaffirming to see that much of the advice I've doled out over the years did, in fact, play out as I've written. When you don't sleep; when you eat erratically; and when you're stressed, your weight will likely rise. When you take good care of yourself, it tends to trend back down.

So, yes. Weight does matter in our power-to-weight sport. But, before you get attached to a certain number, take a few weeks and experiment. Weigh yourself every morning, and record that number along with how you feel (happy, sad, strong, weak, tired, energetic, etc.), what you've been eating, and how you're riding. Be totally objective about it. Nobody else has to see your weight or your notes. Treat it like any other metric, such as air temperature or mph.

(As a side note: Yes, you can use a body-composition scale to determine whether those pounds are fat, muscle, or other, but these scales are notoriously inaccurate. A recent *Consumer Reports* review found that even the best model—when compared to the gold standard, the very precise, laboratory-grade Bod Pod—was off by 21 percent. The worst was off by 34 percent.)

Once you have a handle on how your day-to-day weight fluctuates and makes you feel, start incorporating the following steps to optimize your nutrition and fat burning, and continue the experiment to see how you benefit.

QUANTITY VS. QUALITY

I've been writing about health and nutrition since 1994. I have seen every incarnation of every diet come and go (and come and go again), with various names and promises. South Beach, Atkins, Low-Carb, Smart Carb, No-Carb, Paleo, Vegan, VeganPaleo (or Pegan—and, yes, that's a thing), Gluten-Free, Low-Fat, Raw Foods, Plant-Based, Macrobiotic, Ayurvedic, Ketogenic, Zone, Blood Type, Ph, and on and on and on. I'm going to let you in on a secret.

They all work. I could call a respectable credentialed expert, scan PubMed for research, find decorated athlete devotees, and make a solid case for following each and every one. Would it work for you? Maybe. Maybe not. Or, maybe for a while, and then not, when you couldn't maintain it a minute longer. The thing about diet is that human beings are not test tubes, into which you pour x amount of one substance with y amount of another substance and always get the same reaction. We have different hormones and gut microbiomes and muscle-fiber composition and metabolism and, frankly, psychology, making it far more complicated to determine what actually works for any given person. That is why, at any given period of time, *all* of these have been found to "work."

So, with regard to how much fat, carb, and protein you should be eating, I believe you should start with the basic formula, dividing your daily macronutrient intake into about 40- to 60-percent carbs, 20- to 30-percent protein, and 20- to 30-percent fat. Then, adjust to your liking, based on your personal experimentation. What you really want to focus on is the quality of the food you get, because what all these diets have in common is that they emphasize eating whole, natural, nutritious foods and limiting processed foods that are high in sugar, flour, and/or loads of chemicals and additives and not much else. To get you started, I consulted a few go-to coaches and dietitians for their tried-and-true tips.

ELIMINATE EMPTY CALORIES. This is key if you're riding lots—maybe racing—and trying to drop weight to improve your climbing. You need maximum nutrition with minimal filler. That means cleaning up your diet to avoid empty calories. Skip the chips, cakes, and cookies. It's stuff you already know, but it makes a measurable difference when you do it, because empty calories deliver energy, but it's extremely short-lived, while a whole food with fewer calories will leave you fuller longer. For instance, that Bountiful Blueberry Muffin from your Starbucks? It delivers 350 calories—enough to make a small meal—but will leave you hungry again 10 minutes after you eat it—if you're ever satisfied at all. One cup of chopped broccoli, on the other hand, delivers 30—yes, just 30—calories. That means you can make it rain broccoli crowns all over your dinner plate without putting a dent in your daily diet. And, those cruciferous crowns will fill you up, because they're rich in fiber.

"If you are a volume-eater, who likes to see a lot of food on your plate, look for these types of foods that you can eat big portions of for fewer calories," says Leslie Bonci, MPH, RD, sports nutritionist and owner of Active Eating Advice in Pittsburgh. She notes that with the expectation of big portions in today's culture, we are all sort of volume-eaters at this point. Just remember to put portions of protein and fat on your plate to make a real meal of things.

CUT BACK ON THE BEER. You won't hear me telling you that beer (or wine) is empty calories, because I don't really believe it is. While alcohol's health halo may have been sponsored by the adult beverage industry, beer and wine are good sources of antioxidants and, consumed responsibly, are a regular part of many healthy, lean cyclists' diets around the world. The key word there is "responsibly." Research shows that we get an average of 16 percent of our daily calories from booze. Once you actually start adding up your empties—at about 150 calories a pop for beer—it's easy to see how. "That six-pack may go down easily on a Saturday, but it may also fill you out, without making you feel full for any extended period of time," Bonci says.

KEEP THE CARBS—AND BOOST THE FIBER. Carbs have been widely vilified, but if you want to put the power down, especially for watt-sucking efforts like hill climbing, you need to keep your carbs up, says exercise physiologist Robert Pickels, who has trained numerous amateurs and pros in Boulder, Colorado. "You need to maintain your glycogen stores to maintain your workout schedule," he says.

Choose carbohydrate sources like sweet potatoes, root vegetables, whole grains, and beans and legumes that are rich in fiber, aiming for about 30 grams of fiber a day—twice what the average American currently consumes. Fiber not only helps you feel full on less food, but also it is a potent weight-loss tool in and of itself, if you're trying to shave weight. In one study, where people were told to either follow a calorie-restricted diet or to eat 30 grams of fiber a day, both groups lost just as much weight and equally improved their blood pressure levels, blood sugar levels, and inflammation markers.

At a bare minimum, you need 130 grams of carbs—520 calories' worth, or the amount in 1 cup of pasta, 1 cup of beans, and a potato—to survive. Your brain alone will use up to 60 percent of that, leaving little left for your hard-working muscles," says Dr. Sims. "Skimping on carbs is very stressful on your body, which raises your cortisol levels, and leaves you more likely to lose muscle and store fat."

As mentioned, whole-food sources of carbs like sweet potatoes and root veggies are your best picks, but you also can say yes to noodles and still not fear the bathroom scale. In a study of more than 23,000 Italians (but, of course), those who reported eating pasta had the leanest waistlines.

SPREAD OUT YOUR PROTEIN. Eat protein at every single meal, especially if you're riding lots while also trying to hit your best climbing weight. Hard training and weight loss both put you in a catabolic state, says Pickels. "Protein is essential to protect from muscle loss." Research shows that people who eat diets that are rich in protein maintain their lean muscle mass—which you need to push those pedals—while they lose weight, as opposed to losing both fat and muscle. But you can only process so much at a time, so piling it on at dinnertime (as many do) isn't very productive. Aim for about 20 to 30 grams at every meal and snack to get the 85 to 115 grams of protein active cyclists need each day (that's about twice the amount sedentary folks need).

EAT FAT, GET FIT. Despite the fact that health officials and even the U.S. government have declared the low-fat dieting trend dead, it remains deeply buried in the minds of millions. A recent Gallup Poll reports that nearly half (47 percent) of Americans are still actively trying to avoid fat in their diets.

"Fat is your friend!" says Dr. Sims. "As a cyclist, you use it to fuel long rides. Healthy fats from fish, nuts, avocados, and olive oil reduce inflammation in the body. And, you need fat to absorb essential nutrients like vitamins A, D, E, and K." So, put the low-fat products back on the shelves, and enjoy the flavor and health benefits of this essential macronutrient. And, *yes*, that includes dairy and salad dressings.

In a paper published in the *Journal of the American Medical Association*, Dariush Mozaffarian, MD, DrPH, and dean of the Friedman School of Nutrition Science and Policy at Tufts University, laid out the follies of fat phobia: "Placing limits on total fat intake has no basis in science and leads to all sorts of wrong industry and consumer decisions. Modern evidence clearly shows that eating more foods rich in healthful fats like nuts, vegetable oils, and fish has protective effects, particularly for cardiovascular disease. Other fat-rich foods like whole milk and cheese appear pretty neutral, while many low-fat foods like low-fat deli meats, fat-free salad dressings, and baked potato chips are no better and are often even worse than full-fat alternatives. It's the food that matters, not its fat content." Words to live by.

EAT TO RIDE: TIMING IS EVERYTHING

Equally important is the timing of your nutrition. If you're trying to lose weight, maintain your ideal climbing weight, or just not gain weight, smart nutrition timing is your greatest ally.

Too often, riders get stuck in a cycle of underfueling their rides, finishing ravenous, and overeating later. Then, they beat themselves up, and repeat the process all over again. Let's stop that cycle. First, a little math.

Depending on your size, you can store 1,700 to 2,000 calories of glycogen in your muscles and liver. Hard, hilly rides can torch up to 800 calories (more if you're going *really* hard) an hour. At that rate, it doesn't take long to drain the tank, and you're going to slow down as it approaches empty. Chances are good, if you're trying to lose some weight or maintain an ideal climbing weight, that you're not starting out on full either, so you're beginning your ride compromised. Even if you're a good fat burner, you'll go faster with enough glycogen on board.

"The best way to shed unwanted pounds and still ride strong is to fuel your workouts and be restrictive during the rest of the day," says John Verheul of JBV Coaching, who advises elite-level cyclocross riders, time trialists, triathletes, and more. Here's how to do that.

KEEP YOUR FUEL TANK TOPPED OFF. Time your carbohydrate intake so you top off your tank before a hard ride and replenish what you've burned right after you're done. When you know you'll be going really hard (a hilly race, interval workouts), fuel up with a carb-rich meal 2.5 to 3 hours before. Something easily digestible like rice with a little chicken or oatmeal with nut butter is good. Then, about 15 minutes before you go, pop a few energy chews to top your tank. For longer, tempo-pace rides, you can eat closer to go time. That means having a 150- to 200-calorie pre-ride snack that will provide sustained energy, such as an apple with peanut butter, some Greek yogurt, or a date-based bar. If you're going to be out for more than 90 to 120 minutes, pack food with you and take in about 150 to 180 calories an hour after that point.

Notice that all those pre-ride meals and snacks include protein. That's key for maintaining your muscle tissue during hard training rides. A study published in *Sports Medicine* shows that pairing protein intake with your hard rides and workouts can improve your body's ability to make muscle out of the protein you eat (an ability that diminishes with age), as well as boost how well your muscles adapt to your training efforts. The end result is that you hang onto the muscle you have and ride stronger and faster for years to come.

Afterward, have ride-appropriate recovery food. If it wasn't a very hard effort, you can simply go about your day. Follow up longer and/or harder rides with food and hydration, including about 25 grams of protein, which will speed muscle recovery. When possible, time your rides so you finish around mealtime. That way, you can just eat as you normally would when you're done. One of my favorite midday riding tricks is the 50/50 meal split, where I'll eat half my lunch as my pre-ride fuel and half my lunch as my post-ride fuel.

REPLENISH ON RECOVERY DAYS. Though you're not fueling rides on recovery and/or rest days, you *are* eating to facilitate recovery so that your hardworking muscles can mend and come back fresh and ready for action. That means plenty of high-quality protein, high-fiber carbs, and healthy fats. Bonci's typical rest day recommendations are whole grain cereal like oats with nut butter and milk and fruit in the morning, a spinach salad topped with avocado and lean protein for lunch, and a lean protein with brown rice and veggies at dinner. Just go easy on the snacks and second helpings.

GO TO SLEEP A LITTLE HUNGRY. If you're looking to maintain fitness while losing weight, go to bed just a little bit hungry, advises Pickels. It's an easy way to lose about a sustainable pound a week.

Speaking of sleep, don't skimp on yours. It will derail your training and weight-loss efforts. Shortchanging sleep puts your body in a constant state of stress, which increases stress hormones, like cortisol, that promote fat storage and make it that much harder to drop stubborn pounds. This effect can be even more pronounced, if you don't get enough sleep while also trying to lose weight, says Verheul. "Cutting calories has already put extra stress [on top of training] on your body. Don't add another, if you can help it, or you risk overtraining symptoms and a lowered immune system," says Verheul, who personally uses a sleep-tracking app on his phone to keep himself mindful about maintaining quality sleep and sleeping conditions.

PACE YOUR WEIGHT LOSS. Gradual weight loss will be less disruptive to your training and ultimately less draining than trying to lose a lot quickly. If you're aiming for substantial weight loss, you have to be okay with the occasional failed workout, says Verheul. "There'll be times when you don't have the fuel to finish or you crack halfway through," he says. "Just be sure to distinguish between training and racing. You can 'cut it close' with your workouts and be a little underfueled. But, if a race or event is important, then give yourself a full tank of gas for it."

RESPECT YOUR TAPER. Speaking of racing, if you have a key race or event, place your weight-loss efforts aside and perform a proper taper. During a taper, you winnow your riding volume in half, while maintaining a little intensity during the week leading up to your event. During this time, you should also be fueling and hydrating as you would during a recovery day, allowing your muscles and energy systems to fully recover and repair as you stock energy into storage. Warning: One day during this glorious process of renewal, you will look in the mirror and spout a few unprintable expletives at the bloated image staring back.

I can attest that this taper-tick phenomenon is never pleasant. I remember standing in my hotel room the day before IRONMAN Louisville, leg grippers sausaging my thighs, thinking, "Really? All those months of training, and I feel like a water balloon." It's all just part of the science of the taper. Your muscles store about 3 ounces of water along with each ounce of carbohydrate, so you can expect to gain 2 to 4 pounds during your taper week. But, since research shows that tapering can improve performance by 3 percent, it's really just potential energy, so you can turn the throttle wide open and blast up those hills (and, yes, your weight will return to normal . . . likely well before you hit the finish line!).

A LITTLE FASTING MAY MAKE YOU FASTER

For decades, cyclists have sworn by fasted morning rides—rolling out the door after consuming nothing more than maybe some black coffee—as a way to fuel up their fat-burning metabolism and shed unwanted weight. Recently, for the first time, a study confirms that exercise before eating may indeed do just that.

In the study, researchers from the University of Bath in the United Kingdom had a small group of overweight men perform 60 minutes of cardio on two separate occasions—once in the morning after a 12-hour fast and another 2 hours after eating a 650-calorie, carb-rich big breakfast, including cornflakes, toast, and OJ. They collected fat tissue samples immediately before and an hour after each session, to check for changes.

The proof was in their genes—specifically two called PDK4 and HSL, both of which are triggered when your body uses stored fat to fuel your activity. When the men were fasted, the expression of these genes increased. When they exercised after eating, both decreased. That means not only are you not just burning more fat during that bout but also you could enjoy long-term fat-burning benefits, explained the co-author, Dylan Thompson, PhD, in a media release. He noted that, when you exercise after eating, your fat tissue is too busy responding to that meal to fire up these fat-burning

⊙ WHAT TO EAT WHILE YOU CLIMB

Climbing takes a lot of energy. Even if you're not drilling it, you'll be working close to—and when it gets really steep, above—your threshold. That makes it hard to eat on every front. It's hard to fish food out of your pockets and stuff it in your face. It's hard to chew and swallow when you're breathing hard. It's hard for your body to digest what you do get down, as most of your blood is being diverted to your muscles because they're busy trying to get your butt up to the summit. Because you're climbing close to your limit, you're pulling fuel from your glycogen stores; if you fall behind on eating, you'll also run out of energy for climbing. At best, that means slowing to a crawl; at worst, that means grinding to a halt.

Avoid dropping the out-of-energy anchor on long, hilly rides by using the flats and the descents to eat and drink. On very long climbs (especially if there are a few very long climbs on the day), you'll also need to fuel during the ascent. This is where candy is handy.

Gummy bears, Swedish fish, jelly beans, some dried fruit, and/or energy chews are good sources of fast-absorbing sugars that will hit your bloodstream quickly and give you the boost you need (mentally and physically) to keep the pedals turning. Aim to take in some simple carbs about a half-hour before a big climb and then every 15 to 20 minutes while you climb. I like to use chews for this. So, if I have a pouch of Skratch Labs energy chews or PowerBar Energy Blasts (my two favorites), I'll pop a couple at the base of the climb. Then 20 minutes later, I'll pop another one or two, and so forth, until I reach the top of the climb. On an hour-long climb, that delivers between 120 and 200 calories of quick energy.

Remember to stay on top of your hydration as well. The fluid sloshing in your bottles on your bike only weighs you down. Once it's in your system, it helps you up the hill by keeping your blood plasma at healthy levels and your core temperature in check. Drain a bottle an hour, more if it's hot.

---

changes. "Exercise in a fasted state might provoke more favorable changes in adipose tissue, and this could be beneficial for health in the long term," he says.

To do it, start on an empty stomach (before breakfast is best because that's when your glycogen stores are at their lowest), ingesting nothing but black coffee or plain tea (which will boost your energy and free up some fatty acids for you to burn), and ride for an hour or two at easy, base-endurance pace. If you want to ride longer, that's fine; just take food with you and start eating at the 2-hour mark so you don't drain your stores and bonk. Perform fasted rides 2 or 3 days a week, or less often, if you're training hard and/or racing regularly.

9 | WHAT GOES UP . . .

... must come down: Whether you're fast and furious or timid and terrified, once you've earned your descents, you need the skills and confidence to appreciate and enjoy them.

▸ **SOME OF THE WORLD'S** most-accomplished climbers in the professional peloton are among the weakest descenders in the bunch. Dreading the descents not only saps some of the joy from the overall climbing experience, but in a competitive situation, shaky descending can negate any gains you've made on the way up. (The willowy, mountain-crushing Schleck brothers, who both got dusted in the 2001 Tour de France by a stocky, but dive-bomb-descender, Cadel Evans, come to mind.)

Of course, you don't need to be a multitime world champion Peter Sagan–style, super-skilled daredevil to actually enjoy a well-earned descent. You simply need to learn (and then practice) proper technique, which is admittedly way easier to say than it is to do for many new riders as well as long-time timid descenders.

When I surveyed readers on the topic, many cyclists who love flying up the hills admitted to riding the brakes all the way down, and many who admitted to hating every pedal stroke against gravity giddily gushed over their delight for plunging down a mountain pass. And, unlike climbing, where it's easy to practice technique and improve, descending often proves far more difficult.

"I'm working on improving my climbing, and I'm a lot stronger than when I started," Tommy Thornton of Santa Monica, California, told me, immediately noting that he's a "terrible descender—I feel a complete lack of control and tend to ride my brakes the entire way down. I'm working to improve in this area, but steep descents are my kryptonite."

That's because speed is scary. Being scared makes you stiffen up. Stiffening up leads to squirrely bike handling. Squirrely bike handling is scary. And, the whole thing becomes a vicious cycle, according to cycling coach Andy Applegate, who says, "New riders often sit bolt upright, because they don't like how they speed up with their hands in the drops. But that's unstable; your weight is too high and too far forward." They also tend to brake too hard and in the wrong places, which ironically makes the descent more dangerous than carrying more speed.

The best way to improve is to dissect the descent and practice your positioning and technique, one step at a time.

STEP 1: START WITH A STRAIGHT DESCENT

You'd never go to a ski resort and drop into a double black diamond trail (steepest) without honing in your skills and building confidence on the blues and the greens. Yet, that's pretty much what we do as cyclists—drop in and wing it. So, let's start from the top (literally!) on a straight downhill stretch where you can work on positioning, get comfortable going fast, and practice safely "scrubbing" (see right) speed. Then, apply the following techniques.

GET LOW. Your goal is to get as close to the Earth as comfortably possible (but please don't sit on your top tube and rest your chin on your stem, Tour de France–style; it leaves no room for error, and it isn't worth the risk unless you're actually in the Tour de France) because the lower your center of gravity, the more stable you'll feel. Start by shifting your weight back on the saddle and putting your hands in the drops, with your elbows bent and tucked in. If you're not pedaling, keep your pedals level to the ground in the 3 o'clock and 9 o'clock position.

This stance not only lowers your center of gravity but also keeps the rear wheel firmly planted on the ground for better traction. You also have better reach and more leverage with your brakes. Yes, you will go faster, because you're more aerodynamic, but you're also more in control. And, because you have a smaller profile, you're also less susceptible to being blown off by crosswinds, which are common on descents.

Your weight should feel balanced on the bike, so that both wheels feel firmly glued to the ground. You may need to experiment a little with subtle shifts to achieve that feeling, but that's what this straight-shot descent is for. On anything steeper than a mild grade, hover your butt slightly out of the saddle to put more weight into your feet and improve your mobility on the bike. Hovering also allows you to use your legs as natural shock absorbers, and you'll be less apt to be bucked about if the road gets rough. The steeper the pitch, the more rearward—even behind your saddle on very steep sections—you want your weight (consider it the reverse of the steep incline position where you're hunkered forward over your front wheel).

SCRUB SPEED. Those two wheels you're balancing on are the most stable with some speed. When you grab fistfuls of brakes, it gets pretty unstable in a hurry. So, practice scrubbing speed without extreme changes in momentum. Your front brake holds the majority of your stopping power—and pitches you forward at warp speed, if you pull it hard in a panic—so, braking evenly is important. Feather both of your brakes, by gently squeezing them for a few seconds, and then releasing. This will modulate your speed while still letting your bike roll. Practice controlling your speed without braking by sitting up a little bit and/or flaring your elbows to catch some wind, which will also slow you down.

LOOK FORWARD. Keep your eyes up, and look down the road to take in the big picture. This way, you have plenty of time to react to imperfections in the road, gravel, debris, or other potential obstacles. Resist the temptation to look directly down at the pavement ahead of your front wheel, because you

🢅 SPEED WOBBLES

Physics is brimming with complex—and for many of us, practically incomprehensible—forces. One vexing cornucopia of such forces is the speed shimmy or wobble that can happen on fast descents. A wobble occurs when something creates vibrating forces in the frame that amplify to the point where the handlebar (and eventually the whole bike) starts shimmying back and forth at high speed. I've only had it happen once—cruising a paved downhill no-handed on my mountain bike—and it was terrifying (thankfully quickly returning both hands to the bars stopped the shuddering).

There's endless debate on the exact forces at work that cause the wobble—coasting at high speed, riding no-handed, riding a long-framed bike, and being tense have all been tossed out as culprits—but there's no conclusive set of circumstances. The most important thing to know is that, while you may ride your entire life and never experience one, they can happen, and knowing what to do if a wobble starts can prevent a crash.

If you feel a wobble starting, stay calm and immediately clamp the top tube between your knees (or even just lean one leg against the top tube). Often that contact is enough to calm the situation and carry on. Brake gently to scrub speed. On very long, smooth descents, some riders will descend with one or both knees in contact with the frame to dampen any vibrations in the frame that may lead to shimmying.

---

won't have enough safe reaction time to your immediate surroundings when you're traveling at that speed.

STAY LOOSE. Tension is the enemy of smooth descending. When you tense up, your grip on the bike becomes rigid, which prevents the bike from flowing naturally beneath you. Use your mental tricks here, such as counting or repeating mantras to quiet your mind . . . and remember to breathe to stay calm and relaxed. Watch your shoulders, especially, which have a tendency to migrate upward when you're nervous. Keep them down and relaxed, and maintain a moderately firm grip on the bars.

STEP 2: ADD A CURVE OR TWO

Let's be honest, if all roads were straight shots with brilliant, wide-open sight lines, nobody would be afraid of descending. It's the swoops, curves, hairpins, S-turns, and varying degrees of arc that can send your stomach sailing into your throat as you death grip the bar, shoulders elevated around your ears, muttering Hail Marys all the way down the hill. Learning the art of carving through corners (even if you never get to the place where you let it rip and rail them) increases your confidence and turns that anxiety into exhilaration.

There are many elements to downhill cornering. But instead of trying to memorize instructions, I've found it helps to bring to mind what you want to achieve. In a nutshell, you want to take the most direct line through a turn while maintaining traction with the road all the way around. Sure, speed is nice. But, good lines and firm traction are where to start.

Begin with the lines. You can effectively straighten out a curve by taking the proper path through it. Set yourself up coming into the turn by entering wide (without crossing the yellow line, *please*). Then, cut straight through the apex (the center of the corner) and exit wide (again, without crossing yellow). Of course, every corner and situation is unique. But that is the gist of how you want to corner—as straight as safely possible.

Now, think about your position. You steer by leaning the bike. But if you lean both your body and the bike, there won't be much weight on your tires. Tires need weight to maintain traction, so you risk sliding out. Instead, you want to think about leaning the bike, while keeping your weight pressing vertically down, Velcroing those tires to the road. You're going to accomplish this by using your levers—namely the outside leg and the inside hand. So, say you're swooshing down into a right-hand bend. You want to put the outside (left) pedal in the 6 o'clock position and push down hard (this is key for great traction). At the same time, you're going to press down on the bars (hands in drops) with the inside (right) hand to lean the bike. The sharper and/or faster the turn, the more you need to lean the bike, and the harder you'll push your

⬈ COMING BACK AFTER A CRASH

No matter how skilled of a rider you are, accidents can (and do) happen. Road rash heals. Bones knit. But, anyone who's ever crashed hard knows that the mental scars are sometimes the slowest to mend. Fear is natural. It's meant to help keep you safe. It can also make it difficult to get back in the saddle and feel the joy that riding provides. As a mountain bike racer, I've had my share of wrecks over the years. I've also interviewed numerous sports psychologists on the topic. And, I can say with certainty, it is 100-percent possible to regain confidence after a crash. Like learning to climb and descend, it just takes time and technique.

GET ANALYTICAL. Crashing is a very emotional affair. It hurts. It rattles your confidence. It strips joy from an activity you love. It makes you feel sorry for yourself. That's all legit—allow yourself to feel all of those emotions. Then, have a little postmortem with yourself, and determine why it happened. Were you going too fast for conditions? Did a rabbit run out in the road? Objectively analyze the scene, and ferret out the culprit or culprits behind the crash. This empowers you, because you can then take steps to calm your mind. If it was a pilot error, you can fix that and avoid a recurrence. If it was a fluke, you can remind yourself of the hundreds or thousands of rides you've taken when that same thing never happened and realize that the odds of it happening again are slim.

FOCUS ON THE CONTROLLABLE. If a crash on a descent has just left you inexorably fearful of descending, you need to occupy your mind with thoughts that you can control until they elbow out the fear. Remember your breathing and relaxation strategies. Focus on the concrete descending techniques you know—get low, scrub speed, position yourself appropriately. Repeat a calming mantra like, "You've got this."

TAKE YOUR TIME. You want to climb right back on the horse, as they say. But, start slow, and let yourself get back into the groove, focusing on what you know and can control to help convince your stubbornly fearful reptilian brain that it's okay.

levers. Your outside foot anchors your bike, while the inside hand controls the steering.

Very important: Look where you want to go. This is the hardest, yet most important, point, for many nervous descenders. There are so many places they don't want to go—off the road, into the guardrail, into a pothole—that they inadvertently stare at them. Your bike follows your head and eyes because where your head and eyes are pointed, your shoulders and hips tend to be pointed, as well. You want it all to be pointed past the bend in the road and through the exit of the turn! So, look that way.

Now, let's talk speed and control. Even the best descenders need to scrub some speed coming into corners. The difference between them and not-so-good descenders is that they know when and where to scrub that speed. Too often, riders wait until they're in the heart of the turn to decide to hit the brakes. Bad idea. Remember, you turn by leaning. When you hit the brakes, your bike naturally sits up, which makes it considerably harder to navigate the turn (and may potentially send you exactly where you don't want to go). Ideally, you want to modulate your speed ahead of the bend, so, once you hit it, you're carrying a speed you can maintain through it, and pedal out of the exit. Realistically, there will be times when you need to feather the brakes in the bend, especially at first. But, with practice, that should happen less and less.

It may be stating the obvious, but it bears a mention. When it's wet, silty, or otherwise slippery or slick, you cannot corner with the same speed as you would in bone-dry or grippy conditions. Slow down more than usual coming into the corner, and keep the bike as upright as possible through it. You'll be slower, of course, but you'll be upright.

STEP 3: PERFORM REPEATS

The very same riders who will gleefully put themselves in a tunnel of hurt performing hill repeats *up* the mountain to improve their fitness rarely devote the same level of attention to what they're doing coming down the mountain to improve their technique. I'd argue that they should, even if they don't care about going fast downhill, as the skills you stand to gain from practicing on the same descent will help you remain relaxed on downhills, in general, which serves to give you more energy for climbing overall.

I force myself to do this at least once a year at a crazy local century called 2-5-10, which does 10 laps of a 10-mile loop that connects our three hardest downtown hills, 2nd, 5th, and 10th streets. I rarely do the entire thing (though I have twice), but generally hop in for a few laps. The trickiest descent, by far, is the first, coming down the backside of 2nd Street. The first time down, I'm always a little tentative around the bumpy S-turn midway through and the sweeping U-turn at the bottom. It amazes me how at ease and comfortable (and faster) I am after just a few runs through.

It's a technique that works for even the most gravity-leery riders, as Philadelphia-based women's cycling advocate Michelle Lee will attest. To overcome her fear of going with the flow, she rode down the same "damn downhill" 40 times! "I started out as a very timid descender," she recalls. "I was living in Palo Alto, California, at the time. I decided I was going to ride the same descent in the Foothills three times a day, one day a week until I could do it without brakes. I got to know each and every bump and crack and off-camber bit. Each run, I stretched out how long I could go without braking. By the end, this descent and I were friends. And every other descent in the world felt like a potential friend—or partner in crime—too."

Lee is quick to note that she never went, and still does not go, outside of her comfort zone, but the deliberate practice simply extended that comfort zone. "I learned how to really look down the road—in this case two turns out, instead of one—to fully set up the best lines. Also, bike fit matters a *lot* in high-speed descending," Lee says. As a petite rider, she's too stretched out on many traditional frames and enjoyed remarkable improvement after getting a custom bike that fit her properly. "There is a *huge* difference carving in the turns and being able to work the brakes, as needed," she says.

This is a good place to emphasize the importance of a good bike fit. I've seen many a rider bemoan their lack of ability when, in fact, they're fighting the physics of an ill-fitting bike. Fit factors like too much or not enough weight on your hands can be the difference between bombing down a descent or just plain bombing a descent. A stem that is too long or too short; bars that are too high or too low or too wide or too narrow; a saddle that is too far forward or rearward all impact how your bike rides and responds and ultimately descends. While you're at it, remember to practice adjusting your tire pressure—another big factor, along with tire width in how well you can grip and rip as the pavement plunges down the hillside. It takes a little time and attention, but the rewards are totally worth it.

10 | SMALL BUT MIGHTY

Kickers and punchy climbs may not be very big, but if you're not careful, they can really knock you out.

▶ **BIG MOUNTAINS GET ALL** the glory, but anyone who's ever ridden across the country will tell you that it's not the towering Rockies that break you, but the relentless rolling hills of states like West Virginia and Pennsylvania. In fact, when I surveyed a few hundred riders on their most vexing climbing questions for this book, the vast majority had nothing to do with the 10-plus-mile monsters you'll find in the following chapter, but instead focused on managing short, punchy climbs.

Nearly everyone echoed the same sentiments. "Love long, steady climbs. Hate short, steep climbs." "Love long, sustained climbs. Not so much on the shorter kickers, especially when consecutive for hours on end!" "The longer the better, but long and gradual. Those 20 percents I just can't do!" "I ride where there are lots of steep climbs of varying lengths. It's so difficult to tackle one after another. What's the best way to approach this kind of terrain?"

ANATOMY OF A HILLY RIDE

To understand just what makes bumpy terrain such a beatdown, it helps to peer inside your physiology to see what's happening.

WATTAGE DEMAND: By now, you know that successful climbing is rooted in correct pacing, or how you meter out your efforts to make it to the top. That's all well and good on a long, moderate climb. But what often happens in the hills is that you hit a 10-percent grade or higher right out of the gate, and sometimes, it stays that way for the better part of the climb. That demands watts—lots and lots of watts.

A few years ago sports physiologist Allen Lim, PhD, founder of Skratch Labs, pulled together a physics-based formula for a quick hack for calculating how many watts it takes to get up any given hill:

$$\text{Bike + Rider Weight (kg)} \times 9.8 \times \text{Elevation Gain (meters)} / \text{Time (seconds)} = \text{Power (watts)}$$

Then, tack on 10 percent to account for friction and air resistance.

For example, let's look at my fastest time up the steepest, hardest hill in my backyard—Tenth Street over South Mountain. According to Strava, it's 0.8 mile long, with an average grade of 8 percent and a brief bar-chewing max of 26.1 percent halfway through. Here's how that plays out, according to Dr. Lim's equation:

69.5 kg for my bike and me

122 meters (400 feet) elevation gain

351 seconds (5:51 minutes)

69.5 × 9.8 × 122 / 351 = 237 watts + 24

So, the grand total is 261 watts. Now consider that my functional threshold power (FTP) is 240. I've just gone about 10 percent over my threshold power for about 6 minutes. Recalling our discussion on "matches" in Chapter 3, I haven't really burned a match, but I've played with fire. The steep nature of many hills leaves a rider with few options, even if you're trying to be as conservative as possible.

MAXED-OUT MUSCLE FIBERS: Producing the power it takes to conquer steep ascents—say anything in the 15 percent range and above—is akin to lifting weights as you push the pedals with all your force to propel you and your bike forward up the incline. So, just like when you get in the leg press machine and start pushing the sled, your muscles burn up their adenosine triphosphate (ATP) stores, which are their main source of energy, very quickly. You need oxygen to create more, and that's in short supply when you're huffing and puffing on a vertical incline.

GLYCOGEN STORE RAID: Fully loaded, you have between 400 and 500 grams, or about 2,000 calories' worth, of stored glucose and carbohydrates (glycogen) at your disposal. About 85 percent of that is stored in your muscles. The rest is stashed away in your liver. Lab tests conducted by Iñigo San Millán, PhD, of the University of Colorado Sports Medicine and Performance Center in Boulder, find that you burn about 1 gram a minute just riding along, about 2 grams a minute at endurance pace, and about 3 grams a minute at race pace. Since race pace and climbing pace are both around your threshold, you can expect to decrease your glycogen stores pretty quickly on a hilly ride. Climbing out of the saddle increases that energy use by about 10 percent and drains your power pantry even more quickly. Burning matches also burns lots of glycogen. Research shows that you use energy about 10 percent faster when you're pushing above threshold.

BRAIN DRAIN: Speaking of glycogen, your brain burns about 120 grams of glucose a day, even if you're doing nothing more strenuous than watching *Seinfeld* reruns. That's like two Hershey's Kisses an hour. Now, throw in a steep climb? Crank up the chocolate factory, especially if you tend to get anxious and nervous going into uphill stretches, which wastes precious energy that you're going to need later.

And that's just one climb. Depending on the ride, you could have a

(continued on page 130)

HILL TRAINING SECRETS OF THE FLATLANDERS

A little while back, I raced the Hilly Billy Roubaix,

a West Virginia early summer event that includes nearly 8,000 feet of gnarly climbing over 75 miles of roads that make oxcart paths in Brazil look like the Autobahn.

I spent most of the day jockeying back and forth with this muscley guy in a black kit dotted with midsize flamingos. "Nice kit!" I said to him during a rare moment where we were both breathing easily enough to converse.

"Thanks. I'm from Miami," he replied. "Gotta represent."

Another rider who'd been dangling on our little pack was aghast. "How do you train for *this* down *there*?!"

Mr. Flamingo replied coolly, "Eh... watts is watts."

Indeed. There's no shortage of stories of flatlanders who tailor their training to get the adaptations they need for conquering climbs. Take professional triathlete and coach Aubrey Aldy, who regularly races hilly Ironman events in destinations like Lake Tahoe, California, and Lake Placid, New York. Like others in pancake-flat, windswept states, Aldy told *Bicycling* magazine how he uses all that air resistance to his advantage. His drill: Figure out what direction the wind is coming from and ride 2-mile intervals into it at between 60 and 70 rpm, with a long recovery of 2 to 3 miles of easy spinning. Repeat three or four times. If the wind isn't blowing, Aldy says he just hops on his trainer for this workout: a 20- to 30-minute warmup followed by 8 x 1-minute intervals at 50 to 60 rpm and 125 percent of threshold power (it should feel like an 8 on an effort scale of 1 to 10). Spin easy for 4 minutes between each interval.

Or get *really* creative like Eric Barton of Fort Lauderdale, who shared an epiphany he had one day after getting his rump handed to him in the hills of Asheville, North Carolina. The story he shared with *Bicycling* is so good, I'll let him tell it in his own words from here.

"We're halfway up to the Five Points trail intersection in the mountains outside of Asheville, and I'm certain this hill is trying to murder me. My college buddy Jeff Keener—a local who helps to maintain the trails in the Pisgah area—yells encouragement from up front. But, this Florida flatlander just can't pedal on.

"We circle back down to the lower Bent Creek trails in an air of defeat. When I get home to Fort Lauderdale, I vow to scale the hills next time. But, in a place where landfills are the tallest peaks, how do I prepare? One afternoon, I ride by a parking garage—and inspiration strikes.

"Just after sunrise the following Sunday, I steer my road bike downtown, where there are at least 20 multilevel garages. A county-owned garage is first, with its low-gear ramp up to the second level. The garage evens out after that initial ascent, and by the top, I'm barely puffing. I realize that I'll need multiple garages—10 or more, at least—to make this a decent training regimen.

"I learn some other important lessons on this first outing. Garages in the entertainment district serve as bathrooms on Saturday nights. Some office garages are dusty traps full of stale exhaust. In another, a parking attendant chases me down on a golf cart. It becomes clear that the ideal garage is relatively clean and well-ventilated, has steep-enough ramps to offer a heart-pumping challenge, and lacks aggressive security. Low traffic is also a must, as cars simply aren't looking for bikes around 90-degree turns—luckily most office garages remain empty on weekend mornings. Soon, I'm mapping out alternate routes and bragging about a new hillclimb regimen.

"Now, a year later, a group of us regularly ride what we call the Tour de Garage, bombing through downtown Fort Lauderdale on weekends, before the midmorning brunch traffic hits. At the hospital garage, "My Morning Jacket" blasts from a

(continued)

HILL TRAINING SECRETS OF THE FLATLANDERS (CONT.)

portable speaker stuffed into a bottle holder, echoing off concrete as we corkscrew up seven stories, a constant practice in out-of-the-saddle climbing. At the top, the sunrise paints the skyline a majestic orange. And, then, we scream down, hitting county road speeds, turning tight around the pylons.

"From the quiet streets, we launch ourselves into the library garage—its long, flat levels connected by steep ramps, creating a practice in downshifting and a test for thighs and calves. A dozen garages later, our Strava maps look like doodles, a series of squiggly circles showing ascents. We climb more than 700 feet in 13 miles. This interval training makes our heart rate charts jog up and down like mountain ranges.

STATS FROM ONE SUNDAY TOUR DE GARAGE

- Sea-level garages conquered: 12
- Average stories climbed per garage: 5
- Peak heart rate: 178 bpm
- Top descent speed: 31 mph
- Total elevation gain: 720 feet in 13 miles

"Security guards sometimes eject our group of middle-age bicyclists, and occasionally, we wipe out around turns. But, the Tour de Garage is the type of ride where you hear your buddies laughing all the way around corners, and you take selfies at the top—calves burning, chests thumping, another building conquered. I'll head to Asheville soon, and hopefully, make it up to Five Points."

---

dozen—or more—lying in wait. Much of the advice from the earlier chapters will help, of course. Shift gears early and often, and try to spin more than mash to stay aerobic and put your muscle fibers under less duress. Add plyometrics and heavy strength training to your repertoire so you improve your muscle efficiency and have more muscle fibers at your beck and call. Whatever you do, don't make matters worse by panicking. Break up the climb into manageable chunks. Belly breathe. Count your pedal strokes. Keep calm and climb on.

You can also incorporate some hill-specific training and techniques into your routine to improve your ability to push hard up power climbs.

GET HILL STRONG

I do a lot of mountain bike stage races, where you have mammoth hour-long climbs, short, stem-chewing grinders, and rollers all thrown into the mix, for 4 to 6 hours a day, day after day. When I started, I couldn't force myself to do what I needed to do to succeed at grueling mountainous multiday mountain bike stage races like ABSA Cape Epic and Brasil Ride, so I hired coaches to dish out what I knew I needed most—hill repeats and lots of them.

Yes, it's *way* more fun to just do a hilly ride, but there's a specificity to hill repeats that works like nothing else. For one, you can really dial in your time at intensity—a key factor for hill-climbing success. So, when my teammates and I would do 3 x 8-minute or 6 x 5-minute hill repeats, we would have 24 to 30 minutes at threshold (where you naturally climb). To mimic real-world conditions, where you're hanging onto attacking riders or trying to stay away or make a break, we'd also do multiple short, super-punchy hill repeats like 8 x 3 minutes or 12 x 2 minutes—so the same time at even higher intensity. These not only train your body to produce more power aerobically, better manage lactic acid, and produce more power at your threshold but also bolster your mental reserves, because it's just as challenging for your mind to blaze up the same lung-busting climb as it is for your muscles.

The following hill repeats will address all your hill-climbing needs. You'll find them worked into the plans in Chapter 12, or you can just sprinkle them into your existing riding regimen. For the best results, do one of these workouts once or twice a week on fresh legs. Also, though hill repeats are designed to be somewhat torturous, they're not intended to bury you. Your speed, intensity, and/or power should be within the goal range on every

(continued on page 134)

TEST YOUR METTLE: FIVE STEEP HILLS IN THE STATES

The big mothers in the next chapter steal the destinations spotlight, but there are some insanely hard hills that deserve a place on the stage of must-ride spots. Here are a few my colleague Molly Hurford and the editors of *Bicycling* magazine rounded up to put on your bucket list.

CANTON AVENUE, PITTSBURGH

The steepest paved street in Pittsburgh—and one of the toughest climbs in the U.S.—makes the top spot on the list. Its gradient maxes out at 37 percent, and the pavement is broken and cobblestoned along its 630-foot length. You earn truckloads of bonus—and bragging—points if you do this one as part of the Dirty Dozen, Pittsburgh's annual 50-mile race, which includes 13 of the city's gnarliest climbs (including some cobbles—and very often, crappy late-November weather—for an added challenge).

- Length: 630 feet
- Elevation Gained: 106 feet
- Average Gradient: 13 percent
- Ride It: strava.com/segments/839155

FARGO STREET, LOS ANGELES

The shortest climb on our list is almost as steep as Canton Avenue in parts. It will take only a few pedal strokes to power to the top—if you are strong enough to avoid stopping and walking.

- Length: 330 feet
- Elevation Gained: 154 feet
- Average Gradient: 34 percent
- Ride It: strava.com/segments/9137662

APPALACHIAN GAP, STARKSBORO, VERMONT

This iconic New England climb can be approached in a few ways, but at 2.4 miles long and an 8-percent average grade, the western ascent is arguably the most brutal. Compared to 30-plus percent, that might not sound tough—but have no doubt, it's steep.

- Length: 2.6 miles
- Elevation Gained: 1,153 feet
- Average Gradient: 8 percent
- Ride It: strava.com/segments/295

BRASSTOWN BALD, HIAWASSEE, GEORGIA

Brace yourself for this climb, because it gets steeper the closer you get to the top. The South is not known for its climbs, but Brasstown Bald is one of the greatest. It is well worth the extremely painful 2.4 miles at an average grade of 11 percent so that you can enjoy the view at the top of the climb.

- Length: 2.4 miles
- Elevation Gained: 1,376 feet
- Average Gradient: 11 percent
- Ride It: strava.com/segments/614827

PLATTE COVE ROAD, WEST SAUGERTIES, NEW YORK

Otherwise known as Devil's Kitchen, it's a tough climb that gained notoriety during the 1990 Tour de Trump, when several pros were forced to get off their bikes and walk stretches of it. For New York City residents, it's an easy-to-get-to weekend ride spot and well worth the trip, if you're hoping to crush your competition in climbs on group rides.

- Length: 2.3 miles
- Elevation Gained: 1,249 feet
- Average Gradient: 10 percent
- Ride It: strava.com/segments/252411

repeat. If either drops off by 20 percent, you're close to cooked, and it's time to spin easy and call it a day. Always warm up for about 15 minutes before launching into intervals and cool down for a few minutes when you're done.

UPHILL SPRINT 20S

Being able to surge and recover helps you hang with the group up punchy climbs and gives you the reserves to power through undulating climbs that kick up into double-digit grades.

DO IT: Find a hill that takes 10 to 15 minutes to climb. Start climbing at your lactate threshold (Zone 4/RPE 7 to 8). After 2 minutes, stand up and attack at just below all-out sprint intensity (Zone 5/RPE 9) for 20 pedal strokes. Sit and go right back to climbing at your LT. Repeat every 1 to 2 minutes (depending on your fitness) all the way up the hill. Perform the drill one or two more times.

ROCK THE ROLLERS

To keep going strong through rolling terrain, practice 2-minute attacks.

DO IT: Find a short climb or series of climbs that takes about 2 minutes to crest. Wind up before you hit the climb, so you're at LT (Zone 4/RPE 7 to 8) as soon as the hill starts. Climb at LT for 90 seconds, then go as fast as you can (Zone 5/RPE 9 to 10) for the final 30 seconds all the way to the top. Repeat four to six times.

SHORT-REST REPEATS

These classic climbing intervals simulate real-world climbing conditions where you often don't have the luxury of fully recovering before you're hit with the next incline.

DO IT: Find a climb that takes about 10 minutes to climb (it can be longer, you'll just be turning around before you reach the top). Roll into the climb and crank your intensity to your LT heart rate and/or power (Zone 4/RPE 8). Hold it there for 6 minutes. Flip around and recover for 3 minutes. Repeat for a total of four climb intervals. Alternately, you can perform these as 3 x 8-minute climbs with 4 minutes of recovery.

ROCKET DRILLS

As the name implies, these short intervals go from 0 to 60, like a rocket, to develop the explosive strength and power you need to punch up steep climbs without losing speed and momentum.

DO IT: Find a short incline that takes about 2 minutes to crest. Begin from a standing or slow-rolling start (much as you would a race), on a count of three, explode up the hill as hard as you can (Zone 4 to 5) for 2 minutes. Recover for 5 minutes. Repeat 5 to 10 times.

ONE INTERVAL TO RULE THEM ALL

Because no hill is exactly the same, the best hill-training workout conditions your body to be ready for whatever the terrain tosses your way. That's why I occasionally like to roll all the intervals into one real-world suffer session. My general philosophy is climbing workouts should be hard—stupid hard. That way, when you're out on the road, it's that much easier to fly up the mountain any which way you like.

The three-stage hill-attack plan (pages 138 to 139) targets all your climbing muscles and energy systems. It's designed to improve your muscular endurance to withstand the sustained wattage output that long climbs demand; boost lactate threshold so you can maintain harder efforts without blowing up on the short, steep stuff; and build your aerobic engine so that you can keep your cadence relatively high to avoid frying your muscle fibers with undue stress.

(continued on page 138)

🞧 TOE THE LINE

Even if you don't like to race, you should consider lining up for just one hill-climb event.

You don't need a team. There's really no fear of crashing (though toppling over at slow speeds has been known to happen). It's really just you against the mountain, and a sea of camaraderie. Here are a few marquee events, compiled by *Bicycling* magazine contributor Evelyn Spence, to consider.

MT. TAMALPAIS HILL CLIMB, STINSON BEACH, CALIFORNIA

This 50-year-old race—which brings in 350-plus riders every September—begins with 4 miles of flats along Bolinas Lagoon before rearing up the 4-mile, 1,500-foot ascent on Bolinas-Fairfax Road. The kicker? The last 4 miles offer ever-punchier rollers, officially known as the Seven Sisters—or sometimes the Seven Bitches.

- Miles: 12.2
- Elevation Gain: 2,200 feet

SUNSHINE HILL CLIMB, BOULDER, COLORADO

Sunshine Canyon begins in Boulder and tops out at the historic mining town of Gold Hill. Every May, intrepid amateurs line up next to the town's numerous pros. Grades average 6.7 percent on the first half of the climb but surge up to 14 percent in spots. There's a respite that includes flats and a descent before riders hit washboard gravel with switchbacks purported to reach 23 percent—where it's time to either push on, or blow up and turn back.

- Miles: 9.1
- Elevation Gain: 3,226 feet

MOUNT ASHLAND HILL CLIMB BIKE RACE, ASHLAND, OREGON

Thirty years ago, a couple of roadies challenged a couple of mountain bikers up Mount Ashland from Lithia Park. The roadies took paved Highway 99. The others followed dirt roads past mineshafts and ponderosa pines. They met on the last 2 miles before finishing at the local ski area (6,500 feet). No one remembers who won, but the question of superiority is revisited every September.

- Miles: 18 (dirt), 24 (road)
- Elevation Gain: 4,600 feet

GEAR UP FOR LYME MOUNT EQUINOX UPHILL BIKE CLIMB, MANCHESTER, VERMONT

Scheduled 2 weeks before the legendary Mount Washington Auto Road Bicycle Hillclimb (see page 151), this ride up the highest peak in southern Vermont's Taconic Range is the perfect tune-up for those compact cranksets. It's just as steep, but shorter by a few miles and far less windy. Families cheer for riders along the route, and prizes include stays at local B&Bs.

- Miles 5.4
- Elevation Gain: 3,248 feet

TETON PASS HILL CLIMB, WILSON, WYOMING

Highway 22 traverses an 8,431-foot gap between Jackson's outskirts and Victor, Idaho. In winter, the summit parking lot is packed with backcountry skiers; all summer, cyclists try to outcrawl each other up its exposed 10-percent grades—which alternate with short, lulling flats—for glimpses of the Teton Range. Once a year, in July, you can throw down 20 bucks, meet at Hungry Jack's General Store, and join the official competition.

- Miles: 4.7
- Elevation Gain: 2,284 feet

If you're new to riding intervals, go through it just one time. After a couple of weeks, you can add another round. If you're already an interval veteran, you can jump in and do two sets out of the gate.

These are best performed on a steady climb that's about a 5- to 8-percent grade. Always warm up for 10 to 15 minutes beforehand and cool down when you're done. Do these intervals once or twice a week on fresh legs.

STAGE 1: SIT AND SPIN

This part of the workout helps develop your aerobic capacity, so you can rely on your cardiovascular system to help you climb instead of muscling your way to the top, which fatigues you faster.

DO IT: Shift into a gear that allows you to spin at a relatively high cadence (aiming for about 90 rpm, if possible). Maintain that cadence for 5 minutes at Zone 4/RPE 8. (As you progress, gradually extend the time of the interval until you are maintaining it for 10 to 12 minutes). Recover for 3 to 4 minutes. Move to Stage 2.

STAGE 2: POWER SURGE

As mentioned earlier, the punchy nature of hill climbs often pops riders, because it forces them into the red without adequate recovery. This interval helps to develop more power at your threshold, so you'll be better conditioned to handle changes in pitch and intensity.

DO IT: Start climbing at an intensity that is just under your threshold (Zone 3/RPE 6). After 3 minutes, push your pace/intensity so that you're right at threshold (Zone 4/RPE 8). After 2 minutes, push your pace so that you're above threshold (Zone 5/RPE 9). Hold for 1 minute. Recover for 5 to 6 minutes. Move to Stage 3.

STAGE 3: FULL-THROTTLE CHARGE

There are times when you need a bit of turbo boost to power through a steep switchback, crest a climb without getting dropped, or beat your buddies to the top. These max-effort drills accomplish that.

DO IT: Climb at a pace that is at threshold (Zone 4/RPE 8). When you're ready, attack and push as hard as you can (Zone 5) for 10 to 20 pedal strokes (10 to 20 seconds). Back down and recover for 10 to 20 seconds. Repeat four more times. Recover for 10 minutes, and repeat the three intervals from the top, if you're so inclined.

PACING AND TECHNIQUE

Your ultimate goal is to finish a climb as strong (or stronger) than you start it. For most riders, that means starting more slowly than they typically do. Discipline yourself to start just below your threshold, increasing to threshold as you settle in and find your rhythm. Try to avoid burning matches by staying within your threshold range or the place where you're breathing too hard to hold a conversation, but you're not gasping for breath. Use your gears to keep your effort steady throughout the climb.

As you now know, you're faster and more efficient when you stay seated. This, however, is most pronounced on more shallow grades of about 5 percent, where researchers have found that, at high-power outputs, you may be up to nearly 4 percent faster staying in the saddle. Once the grade hits about 15 percent, however, all bets are off from a speed standpoint. (Though seated climbing still uses less energy). On the really steep stuff, it comes down to body type and traction. Bigger riders are often best served staying seated, while lighter riders benefit from getting out of the saddle to help get a little help from gravity to keep the pedals turning around.

When the grade gets crazy steep—pushing into the 20 and 30 percent range—you'll need to lean forward toward your bars to lower your center of gravity and, in some cases (especially on bumpy mountain bike or gravel ascents), to keep the front wheel from popping off the ground. In this position, you'll need to also keep weight on the rear wheel by gently pulling back on the bar or even hovering a bit over the back of the saddle. To allow plenty of breathing space, keep a flat back as opposed to hunching forward. Remember to spread the workload around between your lower body muscles by shifting your weight forward and back as you can. Drop your heels slightly to give your quadriceps a bit of a reprieve by bringing more hamstring into the stroke.

Finish the climb with conviction, pedaling up and over the crest and continuing on, allowing your body to recover on the fly, rather than coming to a crawl over the top. It not only flushes your legs for better, faster recovery, but also it is a good habit mentally. You want your visual memory to be of you charging victoriously over the summit, not slumping like a rag doll that's just been pulled from the washer.

11 THERE BE MONSTERS

Looming peaks elicit feelings of awe and fear, pain and suffering, and the chance to slay demons, find religion, and savor the sweet rewards that come from a long, hard fight to the top.

▸ **ARGUABLY THE MOST FAMOUS** climbing quote ever uttered came from intrepid mountaineering legend George Mallory as to why he was setting his sights to the summit of Mount Everest: "Because it's there."

Such a deceptively simple answer that speaks to the complexity inside us all, which drives us to leave the safe, comfortable confines of our chaise lounges and pedal off into the distant cloud-shrouded peaks, knowing full well that it's going to be hard, and it's going to hurt, and we might get cold and wet or hot and dehydrated—or both. We crave the challenge because it's there, because we know joy is the flip side of suffering, and we will find both en route to and upon reaching the summit. In a culture where so much of our reality is of the virtual sort, climbing a raw, steep, very real mountain puts us squarely out in the elements and deep within our physical selves all at the same time. "Because it's there" embodies every reason for every single one of our climbs—because what else would we do?

Cyclists don't ride up Mount Everest, of course (though if you go to page 171, I'll tell you how to create your own Everest wherever you ride). We do, however, seek to bag our own towering peaks, whether they be in far-flung locales or in our own backyards. Here are 10 bucket-list worthy climbs right here in the states and some fun facts, training advice, and gear tips for each.

LE MAUNA KEA, HAWAII

Climbing aficionados agree that this mammoth volcanic monster is indeed the hardest climb on the planet. It's one of the only climbs that actually starts at sea level (you couldn't ride from the true base if you wanted to because it begins deep under the surface of the ocean). You travel about 43 miles from the start in Hilo to the summit, gaining 13,800 feet. As if struggling to suck in any oxygen at that altitude wasn't brutal enough, the surface turns to moon dust—powdered volcanic rock, Hawaii's version of gravel—about 5 miles from the top. Riders who have completed the route report that the final 5 to 8 miles can take hours, because you're only able to make forward progress at a rate of about 2 miles an hour when you figure in short breaks of walking or stopping to catch your breath. For reference, one Mauna Kea equals about four Alpes d'Huez (one of the most infamous Tour de France climbs). It averages just over 6 percent incline and hits pitches of about 15 percent.

"I've ridden Mount Washington at least 15 times. Mauna Kea on the Big Island is so much harder," says Doug Jansen, 55. "Fatigue, cramping, altitude sickness—all at the same time! I don't know any other place in the world where you can do more net vertical in fewer miles. There's 5 miles of loose cinder above 10,000 feet, at a ridiculous grade. Mount Washington appears as a wee bump compared to Mauna Kea."

If you ride it: Don't try this one out of the gate. Instead, cut your teeth on Haleakala, a perennial favorite among climbers that starts on Maui's North shore. It's still savagely long at 36 miles and 10,000 feet of vertical gain, with panoramic views. But, it's far more manageable, as it's fully paved, and the average gradient is 5.5 percent. You can even do it as a supported event called Cycle to the Sun. If you attempt Mauna Kea, be sure to pay close attention to the following:

- **LAYERS:** It may be 75 degrees at sea level and snowing at the top. You're going to want to pack a jacket and some gloves at the very least.
- **SUPPORT:** Most people who do this climb vigorously recommend doing it with support—have a friend drive a follow car or meet you at various spots along the way. There are very few amenities along the route, so it's nearly impossible to carry all the food, water, and clothes you will need. Plus, if you start getting sick from altitude, you want a reliable extraction plan.
- **ALTITUDE:** You're going to be spending an awful lot of time above 10,000 feet. Be prepared to crawl along at a glacially slow pace and experience cramping, headaches, and all the struggles that come with thin air. Pack layers, and bring extra sunscreen. Research shows that the higher the altitude, the faster you burn. It's hard enough to get to the summit of this thing without getting fried en route.

MOUNT EVANS, COLORADO

Located on one of Colorado's famous "14ers" (mountains that kiss the sky above 14,000 feet of thin air), the Mount Evans Scenic Byway is the highest paved road in North America. People who have climbed Evans on a clear day claim that you can actually see the curvature of the Earth from the top. The entire climb is about 28 miles and tops out at 14,130 feet, gaining 6,590 feet of elevation. Along the way, you pass through three distinct ecosystems and geological formations, including glacial canyons known as cirques, which are amphitheater-like valleys formed by glacial erosion. On paper, the grade of this climb sounds like a cakewalk, averaging just 4.5-percent incline with only a few short stretches that hit 10 percent. But, many regard it as one of the hardest climbs in Colorado, because of the sheer amount of time you spend climbing at high altitude and the fact that you are very exposed for about a quarter of the climb. Mount Evans boasts more time above tree line than any other North American climb. There are a lot of stretches with no guardrails. So, though there's lots of scenery—Denver in the distance; several mountain lakes, including Summit Lake at 21 miles; the Rockies looming to the west; assorted wildlife like bighorn sheep, deer, and white mountain goats—you'll want to keep an eye on the road and your wits about you as you ascend.

If you ride it: You can do Mount Evans as an organized Gran Fondo or road race, which has the advantage of tons of support. The Bob Cook Memorial Mount Evans Hill Climb is one of the longest running, going on 52 years. The race provides mechanical help, feed zones, and drop bags for extra layers for the ride back down. "The altitude is the greatest challenge," says Mark Elsasser who raced it in 2012 on a single-speed. "It really hits you about halfway through. The best part is the descent back to the start—28 mph and very little pedaling," he says. The race also provides a shuttle for those who'd prefer not to descend by bike.

MOUNT LEMMON, ARIZONA

This one's a classic, and if you go, you'll likely be in the company of myriad happy groups of riders, including packs of pros who set up training camps in town for early season, fair-weather miles. Literally thousands of cyclists climb Mount Lemmon every year, and with good reason—while the 28.5-mile distance makes it brag-worthy, it's extremely accessible for climbing enthusiasts of all stripes and shapes. The average grade is just 4.1 percent, topping out in the tough spots at 9 percent, as you gain a total of 6,222 feet of vertical (though pace yourself appropriately; those steeper sections are near the top). Most folks don't bag this one for the boasting rights, though. They come for the stunning scenery. You pedal out in the baking heat of the high desert on the eastern edge of Tucson, which sits at around 2,800 feet of elevation, and zigzag through thousands of iconic saguaro cacti and mesquite trees before the terrain gives way to cooler pine forests. About two-thirds of the way up, you're treated to a visual feast of spectacular rock formations, including the storied hoodoos—thin spires of rock that protrude from arid drainage basins. It tops off at Mount Lemmon Ski Valley, where you'll see some ice and snow year-round.

One of the real joys of climbing Mount Lemmon is descending Mount Lemmon. Unlike many big climbs, which can be exhausting, if not harrowing, to descend (if you're even allowed to ride back down, as some hill-climb events forbid descents), Mount Lemmon is a long, sweeping, joyful, nearly brakeless affair.

If you ride it: Prepare for traffic of all kinds, as Mount Lemmon is a wildly popular destination climb for motorcyclists, cyclists, and motor vehicles. Start off with plenty of fluids—it's the desert after all, and water is hard to find until you hit the town of Summerhaven at the top. Consider packing some cash and stopping for huge fresh cookies at The Cookie Cabin before you head back down.

MOUNT BALDY, CALIFORNIA

If you've ever watched the Tour of California, you've likely seen riders grinding up this leg-breaker en route to the finish at Mount Baldy Ski Area. The climb, which is inarguably one of the toughest climbs in Southern California, is just shy of 13 miles long, with an average grade of 7 percent and a maximum grade of 15 percent, for a total elevation gain of 4,830 feet. This is definitely one of those climbs that lulls you into a false sense of security before it opens wide and shows its razor-sharp teeth near the top. In fact, the first few miles don't feel like much work at all, and it remains pretty moderate along the ridge and through a couple of cool little tunnels. But, once you enter Mount Baldy Village, all bets are off, as the road ramps up to 10 to 14 percent for extended stretches and pitches through multiple tight switchbacks. The sweet spot is where it flattens out some right before it finishes, where you can toss it in a big gear, and crank it to the top.

If you ride it: The top isn't terribly high altitude-wise, but whenever you're ending at a ski area, you have to be prepared for the weather. Remember those layers! And, don't forget to turn on your GPS, so you can see how your performance stacks up against Peter Sagan, Phil Gaimon, Joe Dombrowski, and other top pros on what has become one of the most hotly contended Strava segments around.

ONION VALLEY, CALIFORNIA

This enormous Sierra Nevada ascent with a cute, unassuming name has been billed by many as the most difficult in the state of California to both climb and descend. Because of its sweeping, uninterrupted panoramic views across Owens Valley from the top, it's also been called one of the most magnificent climbs in the world. Onion Valley is 12.7 miles long and averages a 7.8-percent grade with a maximum incline of 12 percent as you climb 5,202 feet to the peak at 9,163. What makes the ascent up Onion Valley Road so daunting is that, from the moment you roll onto it from the white post office in the town of Independence, it never eases up until you hit the paved parking lot at the top. It starts out relatively moderate—4 to 5 percent—and then progressively ratchets up after the first couple of miles, hitting its hardest sections midway through and hovering around an average of 8 percent for the final 10 miles or so, including some steeply pitched, exposed switchbacks. The geography of Onion Valley is unique—it's one of the deepest valleys in the U.S. and surrounded by 14,000-foot snow-capped peaks. It is also a graben, which is a depressed block of the Earth's crust situated between parallel vertical faults. That gives it its extended steep grades.

It's also one of the lesser-traveled climbs, so it can be just you and the mountain, making for a unique experience, says former pro Neil Shirley, who is one of the top climbers in the U.S. "There's no café or visitor center, or even a campground to welcome you at the top; it's just you and your breathless acceptance that it's over; you made it. Because there is nothing but a hiking trail at the summit, there is little vehicle traffic to interrupt your rhythm, which makes for a peaceful, and dare I say, somewhat relaxing time on the climb," he says.

If you ride it: Bring plenty of fluid. It can be extremely hot, especially in the summer months, and there's no place to refill along the way. And, keep your head on the descent. "Coming down will be a whole lot quicker, especially at the higher elevations where the thin air equates to faster descending speeds" with less resistance, says Shirley. "You can go 50-plus mph pretty easily, but be aware of the potential for rocks to be in the road and corners that come up quite fast." Some riders also have encountered wicked crosswinds, making the descent that much trickier to navigate.

WHITEFACE MOUNTAIN, NEW YORK

This towering gem in the Adirondacks is as long and as hard as Alpe d'Huez, and when you crack the lush and fragrant heavily forested sections, equally scenic. At 7.9 miles, it's not particularly long, but the average grade is 8.6 percent, and once you pass through the tollbooth at the beginning of the Whiteface Veterans Memorial Highway, the sucker hits and stays at about 10 percent for 3 miles (this is also where the trees are thickest, so there's not much to look at to distract your mind from the burning sensation coming from your legs). After that point, it tapers off ever so slightly to about 8 percent. The climb dead-ends at a parking lot at the top, where you can hike up 260 feet more to the tippity top, which sits at 4,867 feet, and soak in the panoramic views of Lake Placid, the Adirondacks, and, on a clear day, the skyscrapers of Montreal, Canada, from Whiteface Castle, which houses the visitor's area on the summit. The peak used to be the final climb of one of the stages of the Tour of the Adirondacks. "At the time, I had not done many climbs of that length or duration, so to hit it at the end of a stage after being in the early break all day, made it pretty amazing—and difficult," recalls John Verheul, head coach at JBV Coaching.

"I totally ran out of energy with about 30 minutes to go. Kirk Willet and Tyler Hamilton came by me like I was standing still. I ate a half-dozen doughnuts within just a few minutes of finishing. That was memorable as well. In retrospect, I was inexperienced and not very knowledgeable about the energy requirements for an effort like that. If you're going to go full gas for the better part of an hour, you have to have been eating and drinking really consistently for the earlier part of the ride."

Riders who climb Whiteface *rave* about the descent, which some have deemed the best of any of the top 100 climbs in the U.S. It's posted at 25 mph, but it doesn't take more than a click through on Strava's leaderboards to see riders averaging in the mid-40s and maxing out at more than 50 mph. Not that you *should* do that.

If you ride it: Bring 10 bucks. It's a toll road, so it's $8 to get through (and these things are always subject to inflation). Also mind the hours, which are subject to seasonal change, but generally 8:30 or 9:00 a.m. till 4:30 or 5:00 p.m. You can avoid the toll by riding earlier or later, but you need to get off the mountain before it opens in the morning and before dark in the evening. Or, you can officially race it as part of the Whiteface Mountain Uphill Bike Race, which gives you a nice flattish 3-mile head start into the climb to warm up your legs before you hit the incline in earnest. It might be worth doing just to see the unicycle division participants—and to see if you can beat the one-wheeled wonders, who have spun to the top in as quick as 1:12:57.

PIKES PEAK, COLORADO

If you haven't tackled this one recently, or ever, it's well worth a visit. Not only is this behemoth now fully paved all the way to its 14,115-foot summit but, as of 2013, the whole kit and caboodle is open to unescorted bicyclists (provided you're over the age of 18) year-round. The full distance from the start on Route 24 outside Colorado Springs is just under 24 miles, over which you gain 7,746 feet of breathtaking elevation. The average grade over the entire climb, which undulates quite a bit, is 6.2 percent, with sustained

⊕ HELL, YES, WE CLIMBED THAT!

Jason Sumner, 46, of Crested Butte, Colorado, shares what it was like to ride Pikes Peak with his wife, Lisa, 35.

Pikes Peak is arguably the hardest road climb in Colorado: Roughly 10 miles are above 10,000 feet, and at the summit, there's 40 percent less oxygen than at sea level. In June of 2013, my wife, Lisa, and I decided to climb it.

For the first 6 miles, the smooth two-lane road gently ascended from the mountain's thickly forested floor. But, we kept our efforts in check. Timberline marked the halfway point, where the grade steepened and wind-battered vegetation became sparse. Silent suffering replaced casual chitchat. No need to waste oxygen on small talk.

The final skyscraping miles were the toughest. Some of the upper switchbacks were precipitously steep. Just one hard turn of the cranks spiked our heart rates as we ground up pitches of 10 to 14 percent. Thank goodness for compact gearing.

Around one corner, we thought we spotted the top. But, it was a false summit—1 more mile to go. The wind brought us to a crawl. Any slower and one of us might have tipped over.

After nearly 4 hours, we rolled up to the nondescript summit sign. I leaned over and gave Lisa a big hug—it was her first "14er" summit by foot, car, or bike. It's still one of our most treasured memories.

---

grades of 10 percent and a few bumps that approach 20 percent. The sheer duration at high elevation makes Pikes Peak a contender as one of the most difficult climbs in the world, and certainly in the continental U.S.

Some riders prefer to park at the Crystal Reservoir Visitor Center, which is at just about the halfway mark (and a good spot to refuel, if you're climbing the entire thing), and where the lion's share of difficulty is found. From Crystal Reservoir, you climb 12.5 miles up 4,885 feet, navigating a dizzying (or maybe that's just the altitude) 154 turns over a steady steep grade. This section of seemingly endless switchbacks above the tree line rewards you with glorious mountain views. There are various organized hill-climb events and Gran Fondos up the peak, if you want to do it with support.

If you ride it: Remember that you're in the high mountains, where the weather can change in the turn of a pedal stroke. Lightning is very dangerous at the top, so check for the potential for storms before you go. The summit temperatures can be 30° to 40°F even during the summer. Be prepared with the food, fluid, and layers—spare jacket, hat, gloves, and leg warmers—that you need for this very arduous ascent.

MOUNT MITCHELL, NORTH CAROLINA

At 6,684 feet, Mount Mitchell is the highest peak east of the Mississippi River. This meandering 24.1-mile climb is situated in the Black Mountains. It takes you through thick woods and a series of tunnels as you make your way up to the summit at the dead end of Mount Mitchell State Park road, the highest legal paved road in the eastern U.S. The gradient isn't too taxing, at just about 4 percent average and a 9 percent max. But it's quite long and, like many Southeastern climbs, can be hot and humid.

This is an easy climb to access and tackle on your own accord, but many choose to double-down (or double-up as the case may be) and chalk this one off as part of Assault on Mount Mitchell, which is a 102.7-mile ride from Spartanburg, South Carolina, along the Blue Ridge Parkway to the summit at Mount Mitchell State Park—a total vertical ascent of more than 10,000 feet. The Assault has been going on since the mid-1970s and is one of the best-known centuries in the country.

For the mountain bikers, there's also an Off-Road Assault on Mount Mitchell, which is a 60-mile, mostly off-road bicycle route with 10,500 feet of climbing (so more "vert" per mile for your money). Most of the climbing is on old forest service roads, and you get treated to some fun single track on your way back down.

If you ride it: Plan to register early. The Assault on Mount Mitchell draws a full field of nearly 1,000 cyclists. If you're unsure of the full distance, you can always sign up for the Assault on Marion first. This rolling 74.2-mile ride heads over to Mount Mitchell but doesn't include the final stretch to the top.

POWDER MOUNTAIN, UTAH

There's no shortage of vertical gain to be found in this western wonder filled with spectacular moonscape canyons and mountain ranges. One that stands out, even among the locals, is Powder Mountain on the outskirts of Eden. At just 6 miles, it's not terribly long, but it does gain 3,300 feet in that span, and it *is* terribly steep, with an average incline of 10 percent, a max of 17 percent, and 3 miles that average over 13 percent. Some have called its finishing stretch the hardest in the country outside of Mount Washington. Little wonder it has served as Utah Cycling Association's Hill Climb State Championship.

If a trip up Powder Mountain isn't punishing enough for you, you can try the aptly named "Punisher Ride," which spans 116 miles and racks up more than 10,000 feet of climbing. Because the Powder Mountain descent is steep and fairly straight, and can be insanely (and in a few cases fatally) fast, the Punisher Ride itself ends at the top, and they shuttle you back down. If you go on your own, you do so at your own risk, so be smart.

If you ride it: Take some time to explore the other big mountains ringing Salt Lake City, notably Little and Big Cottonwood canyons, which are not quite as steep but are long, arduous, and, of course, eye-poppingly scenic.

MOUNT WASHINGTON, NEW HAMPSHIRE

No list would be complete (and indeed it's come up multiple times in this book) without the notorious, magnificent Mount Washington, which consistently tops lists of the most difficult hill climbs in the U.S., if not the world. The only word to describe it is "relentless." It's 7.6 miles long, and has an average grade of 12 percent with extended stretches of 18 percent. The last 50 yards snake up 22 percent en route to the welcome center at the summit.

The road is generally closed to bicycles, so the only way to test your mettle up this New England monster is during one of two annual hill climb races (and their designated practice days), the classic Mount Washington Auto

Road Bicycle Hillclimb and Newton's Revenge. The climb begins, somewhat ironically, on a downhill, as riders charge down about a tenth of a mile to the tollgate, where they're immediately greeted by a 12-percent pitch. And, that's pretty much it for the day. The road is thickly tree lined for most of the first half but then opens up to an exposed ridge, where you can see your ultimate destination. About 4.5 miles in, the road turns to well-groomed gravel for about a mile, which is pleasant when dry but can get soft in the rain. When you get to the top, a volunteer wraps you in a commemorative fleece blanket, which is how every hard race should finish.

The weather can be extremely temperamental, with frequent high winds. In fact, until fairly recently, the summit held the record for the highest wind gust not involved in a cyclone (231 mph!). The hill climbs have "weather dates" and are postponed for ice, snow, very high winds, and/or hard, driving rain.

If you ride it: Bring support. Nobody is allowed to ride down Mount Washington. Ever. If you don't have a ride back down, the organizers will not let you ride up. It was so nerve-racking just driving down it, I can't say I'd ever want to even consider trying to pilot a bike down.

CLIMBING INTO RARIFIED AIR

Many of the world's most-famous and infamous climbs take place at elevation, which poses challenges above and beyond the forces of gravity. In short, it's hard to breathe. As elevation rises above 2,000 feet, the air pressure becomes lower, meaning oxygen molecules become more spread out, leaving you with less oxygen in every breath you take. To get the best of these behemoths, you need to be prepared to face the low oxygen and the misery it can bring. I learned to cope with all this the way all great lessons are learned—the hard way.

I can't say that I wasn't warned. My fellow teammates, and even my competitors, gave me their best advice as I headed out to race the Breck Epic, a 6-day mountain bike stage race that was mostly above 10,000 feet. "Don't go into the red, you'll never recover," they said with the gravity of those who had seen things racers don't want to see. So what did I do? Shot off the line like a cannonball, soared into the red, and spent the rest of Stage 1 dropping anchor as everyone in the race passed me by like I was a potted plant.

I learned much from that experience and, following the wisdom of high-altitude experts, I learned even more during two subsequent trips to the infamous races in Leadville, Colorado. Most notably, there's no hiding from or escaping the effects caused by higher elevations, but if you understand what's happening to your body at altitude, you can take measures to prevent the worst of the potential woes and maximize your performance and enjoyment of your next ride into thin air. Here's what's going on . . . and, more importantly, what to do about it.

YOUR BRAIN CRIES FOR OXYGEN

The thinner air generally becomes noticeable as you hit the 5,000-foot mark and pretty much affects anyone by the time you cross into high altitude at 8,000 feet. By the time you reach 12,000 feet, there's a wind-sucking 40-percent fewer oxygen molecules per breath. *Everyone* notices that.

Your brain doesn't like not having enough oxygen, so it sends out the signal to dilate your blood vessels to get more bloodflow and oxygen to the brain. "That's why some people develop a throbbing headache within 30 minutes of arriving at high altitude," says Peter Hackett, MD, director at the Institute for Altitude Medicine in Telluride, Colorado. Ibuprofen is one way to help relieve your pounding head, but to really help your body adjust and get the oxygen it needs before your big event, some experts recommend beetroot juice: It's rich in nitrates that your body converts to nitric oxide, a gas that causes your blood vessels to relax and widen, allowing more blood flow and making it easier to function in low-oxygen environments.

YOUR HEART RATE RISES

Unsurprisingly, your heart rate increases at altitude, as your body compensates for the thinner air. At about 6,500 feet, your heart rate will increase 10 percent over your usual rate at sea level. Heart rate will normalize as you acclimate, but it takes at 2 to 3 weeks to become fully acclimated. If you don't have time to fully acclimate, it's useful to go out for a few of your training rides with a heart rate monitor and recalibrate your heart rate zones for high altitude—then stick to them during race day. (This has worked swimmingly well for me at Leadville, where I learned that burning too many matches will fry you for the day.)

YOUR POWER DECLINES

The same hill you could charge up in the big ring at sea level can leave you spinning in the little ring, still out of breath at high altitude. That's because your power output drops about 3 percent per thousand feet above 5,000 feet elevation. "By the time you hit Leadville and other high-mountain races at 10,000 feet, you're operating at 15 percent less power," says Dr. Hackett. Again, acclimatization helps. But, there's a reason that people who live high often choose to train low—everyone's power suffers to some degree once you hit high altitude.

YOU START TO PEE . . . A LOT

It's not your imagination. You really are running to the restroom (or roadside or trailside) more often at high altitude. It's even got a scientific name—altitude diuresis—and it's actually a wonderful thing. "Your body wants to be a little drier at high altitude. As you pee out some excess fluids, your blood becomes thicker and your hemoglobin becomes more concentrated," Dr. Hackett says.

The cool thing is that this happens within 24 hours of touchdown at altitude, so within a day, you can already carry more oxygen in your blood. "Everyone talks about the dehydration that takes place at altitude like it's a bad thing," he says. "But it's a natural adaptation designed to help you get more oxygen to your muscles and organs." To that end, resist the urge to drown yourself in fluids every moment of every day in the mountains. "You cannot—nor should not try to—completely counteract attitude diuresis," he says. "An extra liter a day is a reasonable amount to stay hydrated without overdoing it."

YOUR APPETITE DECLINES

Some people get nauseated or, in severe cases, even vomit, when they go to high altitude from sea level too quickly. But, even if you don't feel altitude sick, it's natural for your appetite to decline. Research shows that levels of leptin, a hormone known to suppress appetite, increases at altitude. For the best energy and performance, skew your high altitude diet to be higher in carbohydrates, which provide about 15 percent more energy for the same amount of oxygen as you get from fats.

YOU TOSS AND TURN

High altitude can mess up your sleep quality on a few fronts. Most notably, low oxygen directly disrupts sleep centers in your brain, causing frequent waking. You also can experience what is known as sleep periodic breathing, in which (as the name implies) you literally stop breathing for a few moments, and then start up again as the respiratory center of your brain, which senses carbon dioxide, battles with the respiratory trigger in the carotid artery, which senses low oxygen. Both can be quite disruptive to a good night's rest. "Taking a mild sleeping aid like Benadryl can help while you acclimate," says Dr. Hackett.

YOUR BODY STARTS BLOOD DOPING

Getting more oxygen where you need it is priority number one, so along with thickening your blood through a little dehydration, your body will also start producing more EPO—the hormone that regulates the volume and number of red blood cells, so your blood can carry more oxygen—within 24 to 48 hours of your arrival at altitude.

YOUR GENES GO FULL TILT

It can take the better part of a month to fully acclimate to high altitude and, as you may have already deduced, everyone acclimates a bit differently, with some people adjusting relatively seamlessly and others still feeling wheezy and woozy a couple of weeks in. Like so much in life, you can credit (or blame) your personal adaptation process on your genes, says Dr. Hackett. "There are more than 400 genes that are turned on in every cell in your body in response to altitude," he says. "There are also genes that get turned off. You're looking at a tremendous range of gene expression among individuals."

Generally speaking, however, we all fall along a bell-shaped curve, where 60 percent will do about average and take a few days to start feeling better; 20 percent acclimate faster, and 20 percent acclimate more slowly. "No matter who you are, big jumps like sea level to Leadville are too much for 1 day and don't work for anyone. Give yourself 3 to 5 days at altitude before you want to compete or perform well; 7 to 10 days, if you can."

12 PULLING IT ALL TOGETHER: TRAINING PLANS AND CLIMBING CHALLENGES

You're ready to take your riding to the next level, and here's how to get there.

▶ **IT'S EASY TO GET** overwhelmed by all the moving parts in books like this, where we're talking about long rides, intervals, core training, more intervals, strength training, and (are you kidding me?) more intervals. I mean, how the heck does it all fit together in a busy life that includes any combination of work, kids, house, lawn, a healthy social life, and so forth? Relax. The heavy lifting is done for you, so all you have to do is pick a plan, follow along, and get ready to take your climbing (and cycling) ability and fitness to the next level.

TRAINING: THE BIG PICTURE

During base and early season, about 75 percent of your rides should be endurance pace (Zone 2—see page 38 for a training-zone refresher), with the rest including some harder efforts like short intervals, tempo work, and hills. Once the peak riding season is in full swing, and you're out there mixing it up with group rides, races, fondos, and other high-spirited fun, maintain your base by spending about half your riding time performing those endurance-pace (Zone 2) rides. Perform your intervals and hard workouts twice a week. Take at least 1 day a week for recovery.

THE 8-WEEK MY-BASE-IS-BUILT-SO-LET'S-ROLL! HILL-CLIMB PLAN

This plan is designed to elevate your climbing game over a 2-month span. It features moderate volume with a suite of mixed length/intensity intervals to deliver climbing-specific intensity and keep your adaptations coming. You can shuffle days, as needed; just try to maintain the general workload/recovery

MONDAY	TUESDAY	WEDNESDAY	THURSDAY
Rest or X-train/ Core workout	HIIT It: ~60 to 75 mins. with Tabatas (p. 67)	Sustained Effort: ~90 mins. with 3 x 10 mins. Steady State Intervals (p. 43)	Easy Ride: ~60 mins.
Rest or X-train/ Core workout	HIIT It: ~60 to 75 mins. with Full-Recovery Full Throttles (p. 68)	Sustained Effort: ~90 mins. with 3 x 12 min. Steady State Intervals	Easy Ride: ~60 mins.
Rest or X-train/ Core workout	Endurance Ride: ~60 mins.	OFF, full rest day	Endurance Ride: ~60 mins.
Rest or X-train/ Core workout	HIIT It: ~60 to 75 mins. with Uphill Sprint 20s (p. 134)	Sustained Effort: ~90 mins. with 3 x 15 min. Steady State Intervals	Easy Ride: ~60 mins.
Rest or X-train/ Core workout	Ramp It Up: ~60 to 75 mins. with 2 x 20 Ramps (p. 69)	Endurance Ride: ~90 mins.	Easy Ride: ~60 mins.
Rest or X-train/ Core workout	Endurance Ride: ~60 mins.	OFF, full rest day	Endurance Ride: ~60 mins.
Rest or X-train/ Core workout	HIIT It: ~60 to 75 mins. with Power Surges (p. 69)	Sustained Effort: ~90 mins. with 2 x 20 min. Steady State Intervals	Easy Ride: ~60 mins.
Rest or X-train/ Core workout	HIIT It: ~60 to 75 mins. with Ups and Downs (p. 45)	Sustained Effort: ~90 mins. with 2 x 20 min. Steady State Intervals	Easy Recovery Ride: ~60 mins.

pattern. The plan calls for 6 to 9 hours a week. You can certainly extend your rides, if you have the time. The intervals are interspersed to keep the workouts fresh. You'll also enjoy an easier week every third week. Strength training can be added to your interval and/or weekend days. You can do your core workout every day (and should do it at least 2 days a week).

PLAN KEY

Easy Ride: Mostly Zone 1 ride for recovery, tapering, or just enjoying a simple spin in the sunshine!
Endurance Ride: Solid Zone 2, foundation-building rides, often with skills built in.
Sustained Effort: Endurance/Zone 2–paced rides with blocks of tempo (Zone 3).
HIIT It: Endurance/Zone 2–paced rides with high-intensity interval work to build lactate threshold (Zone 4) and VO_2 max (Zone 5) included.

FRIDAY	SATURDAY	SUNDAY
HIIT It: ~60 to 75 mins. with Punchy Ups Intervals (p. 68)	Endurance Ride: ~2 hours, practice technique on any hills	Endurance Ride: ~90 mins. to 2 hours, practice technique on any hills
HIIT It: ~60 to 75 mins. with Hill Charges (p. 68)	Endurance Ride: ~2 hours	Endurance Ride: ~90 mins. to 2 hours, practice technique on any hills
Easy Ride: ~60 mins.	Endurance Ride: ~2 hours with 1 x 20 Steady State Interval	Endurance Ride, practice technique on any hills ~1 to 2 hours
HIIT It: ~60 to 75 mins. with Rock the Rollers (p. 134)	Endurance Ride: ~2 hours, practice technique on any hills	Endurance Ride: ~90 mins. to 2 hours, practice technique on any hills
HIIT It: ~60 to 75 mins. with Big Gear Accelerations (p. 69)	Endurance Ride: ~2 hours, practice technique on any hills	Endurance Ride: ~90 mins. to 2 hours, practice technique on any hills
Easy Ride: ~60 mins.	Endurance Ride: ~2 hours with Short-Rest Repeats (p. 134)	Endurance Ride: ~1 to 2 hours, practice technique on any hills
HIIT It: ~60 to 75 mins. with Extended Bursts (p. 45)	Endurance Ride: ~2:30 hours, practice technique on any hills	Endurance Ride: ~90 mins. to 2 hours, practice technique on any hills
HIIT It: ~60 to 75 mins. with Rocket Drills (p. 135)	Endurance Ride: ~2:30 hours, practice technique on any hills	Endurance Ride: ~90 mins. to 2 hours, practice technique on any hills

THE 12-WEEK I-WANT-TO-CRUSH-THE-CLIMBS-NEXT-SEASON HILL-CLIMB PLAN

This plan is designed to build your fitness and climbing power, starting in the off-season and launching you into the early season. It features moderate volume with a focus on building base and raising your threshold, so you can hang on any incline and still be in the mix at the end of a hilly ride.

You can shuffle days, as needed; just try to maintain the general workload/recovery pattern. The plan calls for 6 to 10 hours a week. You can certainly extend your rides, if you have the time. You'll also enjoy an easier week every third week to help all your hard work sink in. Strength training can be added

MONDAY	TUESDAY	WEDNESDAY	THURSDAY
Rest or X-train/ Core workout	Sustained Effort: ~60 to 75 mins. with 2 x 10 mins. Steady State Intervals (p. 43)	Endurance Ride: ~60 to 90 mins.	HIIT It: ~60 to 75 mins. with Ups and Downs (p. 45)
Rest or X-train/ Core workout	Sustained Effort: ~60 to 75 mins. with 3 x 10 min. Steady State Intervals (p. 43)	Endurance ride: ~ 60 to 90 mins.	HIIT It: ~60 to 75 mins. with Extended Bursts (p. 45)
Rest or X-train/ Core workout	Endurance Ride: ~60 to 75 mins.	Sustained Effort: ~45 mins. with 3 x 5 min. Steady State Intervals (p. 43)	Endurance Ride: ~60 to 75 mins.
Rest or X-train/ Core workout	Sustained Effort: ~60 to 75 mins. with 3 x 15 mins. Steady State Intervals (p. 43)	Endurance Ride: ~60 to 90 mins.	HIIT It: ~60 to 75 mins. with Climbing Intervals (p. 45)
Rest or X-train/ Core workout	Sustained Effort: ~60 to 75 mins. with 2 x 20 mins. Steady State Intervals (p. 43)	Endurance Ride: ~ 60 to 90 mins.	HIIT It: ~60 to 75 mins. with Short-Rest Repeats (p. 134)

to your interval and/or weekend days. You can do your core workout every day (and should do it at least 2 days a week), but it's always scheduled for Monday to get you moving.

PLAN KEY

Easy Ride: Mostly Zone 1 ride for recovery, tapering, or just enjoying a simple spin in the sunshine!
Endurance Ride: Solid Zone 2, foundation-building rides, often with skills built in.
Sustained Effort: Endurance/Zone 2–paced rides with blocks of tempo (Zone 3).
HIIT It: Endurance/Zone 2–paced rides with high-intensity interval work to build lactate threshold (Zone 4) and VO_2 max (Zone 5) included.

FRIDAY	SATURDAY	SUNDAY
Easy Ride: ~45 to 60 mins.	Endurance Ride: ~2 hours, practice technique on any hills	Endurance Ride: ~90 mins. to 2 hours, practice technique on any hills
Easy Ride: ~45 to 60 mins.	Endurance Ride: 2 hours, practice technique on any hills	Endurance Ride: ~90 mins. to 2 hours, practice technique on any hills
OFF, full rest day	Endurance Ride: ~1 to 2 hours, practice technique on any hills	Endurance Ride: ~1 to 2 hours, practice technique on any hills
Easy Ride: ~45 to 60 mins.	Endurance Ride: ~2 to 2:30 hours, practice technique on any hills	Endurance Ride: ~1:30 to 2 hours, practice technique on any hills
Easy Ride: ~45 to 60 mins.	Endurance Ride: ~2 to 2:30 hours, practice technique on any hills	Endurance Ride: ~1:30 to 2 hours, practice technique on any hills

THE 12-WEEK I-WANT-TO-CRUSH-THE-CLIMBS-NEXT-SEASON HILL-CLIMB PLAN (*CONT.*)

MONDAY	TUESDAY	WEDNESDAY	THURSDAY
Rest or X-train/ Core workout	Endurance Ride: ~60 to 75 mins.	Sustained Effort: ~45 mins. with 3 x 5 min. Steady State Intervals [p. 43]	Endurance Ride: ~60 to 75 mins.
Rest or X-train/ Core workout	Sustained Effort: ~60 to 75 mins. with 2 x 20 mins. Steady State Intervals [p. 43]	Endurance Ride: ~60 to 90 mins.	HIIT It: ~60 to 75 mins. with Rock the Rollers [p. 134]
Rest or X-train/ Core workout	Sustained Effort: ~60 to 75 mins. with 1 x 30 mins. Steady State Intervals [p. 43]	Endurance Ride: ~60 to 90 mins.	HIIT It: ~60 to 75 mins. with Uphill Sprint 20s [p. 134]
Rest or X-train/ Core workout	Endurance Ride: ~60 to 75 mins.	Sustained Effort: ~45 mins. with 3 x 5 min. Steady State Intervals [p. 43]	Endurance Ride: ~60 to 75 mins.
Rest or X-train/ Core workout	HIIT It: ~60 to 75 mins. with Tabatas [p. 67]	Sustained Effort: ~60 to 90 mins. with 3 x 8 min. Steady State Intervals	Easy Ride: ~60 mins.
Rest or X-train/ Core workout	HIIT It: ~60 to 75 mins. with Full-Recovery Full Throttles [p. 68]	Sustained Effort: ~60 to 90 mins. with 3 x 8 min. Steady State Intervals [p. 43]	Easy Ride: ~60 mins.
Rest or X-train/ Core workout	Endurance Ride: ~60 to 75 mins.	Sustained Effort: ~45 mins. with 3 x 5 min. Steady State Intervals [p. 43]	Endurance Ride: ~60 to 75 mins.

FRIDAY	SATURDAY	SUNDAY
OFF, full rest day	Endurance Ride: ~1 to 2 hours, practice technique on any hills	Endurance Ride: ~1 to 2 hours, practice technique on any hills
Easy Ride: ~45 to 60 mins.	Endurance Ride: ~2 to 2:30 hours, practice technique on any hills	Endurance Ride: ~1:30 to 2 hours, practice technique on any hills
Easy Ride: ~45 to 60 mins.	Endurance Ride: ~2 to 2:30 hours, practice technique on any hills	Endurance Ride: ~1:30 to 2 hours, practice technique on any hills
OFF, full rest day	Endurance Ride: ~1 to 2 hours, practice technique on any hills	Endurance Ride: ~1 to 2 hours, practice technique on any hills
HIIT It: ~60 to 75 mins. with Punchy Ups (p. 68)	Endurance Ride: ~2 to 2:30 hours, practice technique on any hills	Endurance Ride: ~1:30 to 2 hours, with One Interval to Rule Them All (p. 135)
HIIT It: ~60 to 75 mins. with Rocket Drills (p. 135)	Endurance Ride: ~2 to 2:30 hours, practice technique on any hills	Endurance Ride: ~1:30 to 2 hours, with 1 Ramp Interval (p. 69)
OFF, full rest day	Endurance Ride: ~1 to 2 hours, practice technique on any hills	READY to ROCK!

THE 4-WEEK OH-SH*T-I-HAVE-THAT-HILLY-CENTURY-COMING-UP! HILL-CLIMB PLAN

It happens to the best of us. We sign up for the Heaven's Gate 100 thinking we have all the time in the world to train, and, suddenly, somehow, it's just a calendar flip away. Relax! So long as you've been putting in your base miles, you can channel your inner mountain goat and activate your climbing legs with this emergency 4-week hilly century plan. This plan assumes that you've been riding at least 4 to 6 hours (or about 60 miles) a week. Do the rides when they fit into your schedule, leaving a day of rest, easy riding, or cross-training between your three workout rides.

MONDAY	TUESDAY	WEDNESDAY	THURSDAY'
Rest or X-train/Core workout	HIIT It: ~60 to 75 mins. with Tabatas (p. 67)	Easy Ride/rest/or X-train	Sustained Effort: ~60 to 75 mins. with 3 x 12 Steady State Intervals (p. 43)
Rest or X-train/Core workout	HIIT It: ~90 mins. with Full-Recovery Full Throttles (p. 68)	Easy Ride/rest/or X-train	Sustained Effort: ~2 hours with Short-Rest Repeats (p. 134)
Rest or X-train/Core workout	HIIT It: ~90 mins. with Punchy Ups (p. 68)	Easy Ride/rest/or X-train	Sustained Effort: ~2 hours with One 1 x 20 Interval to Rule Them All (p. 135)
Rest or X-train/Core workout	HIIT It: ~60 mins. with Rocket Drills (p. 135)	Easy Ride/rest/or X-train	Sustained Effort: 90 mins. with 3 x 5 mins. Steady State Intervals (p. 43)

PLAN KEY

Easy Ride: Mostly Zone 1 ride for recovery, tapering, or just enjoying a simple spin in the sunshine!
Endurance Ride: Solid Zone 2, foundation-building rides, often with skills built in.
Sustained Effort: Endurance/Zone 2–paced rides with blocks of tempo (Zone 3).
HIIT It: Endurance/Zone 2–paced rides with high-intensity interval work to build lactate threshold (Zone 4) and VO_2 max (Zone 5) included.

FRIDAY	SATURDAY	SUNDAY
Easy Ride/rest/or X-train	Endurance Ride: ~3:45 to 4:15 hours	Easy Ride/rest/or X-train
Easy Ride/rest/or X-train	Endurance Ride: ~4:15 to 4:45 hours, with hills, practice technique	Easy Ride/rest/or X-train
Easy Ride/rest/or X-train	Endurance Ride: ~4:45 to 5:15 hours ride on varied terrain	Easy Ride/rest/or X-train
Easy Ride/rest/or X-train	HIIT It: ~30 to 45 mins. with 5 mins. Steady State Interval (p. 43) plus 2 Hill Charges (p. 68)	Century!

ZONE CHART

To recap, here are your five basic training zones.

ZONE 1: EASY/RECOVERY
Light and relaxed breathing, barely above normal. You're at 60 to 64 percent of your maximum heart rate (MHR), and less than 55 percent of FTP, if you're using a power meter. You can talk easily. (RPE 1 to 2)

ZONE 2: ENDURANCE/BASE
Deep, steady, rhythmic breathing. This is your aerobic, endurance-training zone, requiring 65- to 74-percent MHR (55- to 75-percent FTP). You can speak short sentences but are starting to breathe more heavily. (RPE 3 to 4)

ZONE 3: TEMPO/INTENSIVE ENDURANCE
Slightly labored breathing. This is a steady tempo pace, requiring 75- to 84-percent MHR (75- to 90-percent FTP). You're working just above your endurance comfort zone—similar to when you're riding with someone who is a bit faster than you. You can speak just a few words at a time. (RPE 5 to 6)

ZONE 4: THRESHOLD/ LACTATE THRESHOLD
Short, fast, rhythmic breathing. This is your lactate threshold zone, requiring 85- to 94-percent MHR (90- to 105-percent FTP). You're hitting your sustainable user limit. It's also known as race pace. You can only speak one or two words at a time. (RPE 7 to 8)

ZONE 5: ABOVE THRESHOLD TO MAX
Hard, heavy breathing. This is your VO_2 max training zone, where you're at 95- to 100-percent MHR (105- to 120-percent FTP). You're utilizing as much oxygen as possible and going as hard as you can. It is impossible to speak! (RPE 9 to 10)

CLIMBING CHALLENGES

Some riders like to meticulously follow training plans and track their every watt and fitness metric along the way. Others prefer to jump in and just ride. Either way, it's nice to have a challenge to keep you motivated and to provide a sense of accomplishment when you're finished. Here are two *Climb!* challenges that will do both.

GET STARTED: THE 2-WEEK *CLIMB* CHALLENGE

If you're generally hill adverse, want to master the finer points of hill-climbing technique, and/or generally new to climbing, this challenge is the place to start. As I've explained, digging into the same climb offers a number of advantages: You can practice standing and sitting at the very same pitches to see which one works best for you; you can work on your shifting and cadence; you can shift your weight and learn how it impacts traction, control, and comfort; and, of course, you can really hone your mental game, as you stare down the same incline for 14 days in a row.

There is only one hard-and-fast rule for mounting your 2-week challenge—you must ride up the same climb every single day for 2 weeks straight. Now, obviously, there are a few commonsense exceptions. If you come down with the flu or there's an ice storm, stay home and reschedule your challenge. Otherwise, I'd encourage you to stick with it, even if it's a little cold or rainy. If you ride long enough, you're going to be caught out in adverse conditions, and it's important to know how to handle them.

Choose your climb wisely. Depending where you live, options may be plentiful or limited, but you want this challenge to be as fun and fruitful as it is sufferable. Ideally, the climb should be long enough to make you work, but not so long that it's unreasonable to make time for it every day. Ten to 30 minutes is a good place to start. Quieter, less-traveled roads make for a more peaceful, contemplative experience. If possible, find a climb with some undulation in the grade, so you can practice on moderate inclines as well as steep pitches. Finally, it's helpful if your climb is reasonably close to home, so you can easily ride to it without taking up too much time in your day.

Recovery will be important during this challenge. So be sure to go into each day well-fueled and have a recovery drink (yes, chocolate milk works) when you get home.

To make the most of your fortnight foray, I recommend assigning a special goal to each ascent. On the following pages, you can see what a sample 2-week *Climb!* Challenge could look like.

DAY 1

Just ride and record it. The first time up your climb, don't change a thing. Go out to that hill, and make your way up it as quickly and as comfortably as possible. Record your time and perceived exertion. Make note of your positioning on the bike as well as your cadence. If you use a heart rate and/or power meter, capture that data as well.

DAY 2

Change your cadence. If you tend to be a masher, try some easier gears and spin a higher cadence. If you're a high-speed spinner, try some power-climbing in a harder gear. Get a feeling for how your heart rate changes and how your leg muscles respond at different gearing and cadences.

DAY 3

Perfect your body positioning. Pay super-close attention to your body positioning today (refresh your technique on page 28). Are your shoulders down and relaxed? Is your chest open? Are your feet flat? Perform a head-to-toe check every few minutes to dial in your perfect climbing posture.

DAY 4

Shift your weight. Play around with your body-weight placement today. Shift your butt forward and back to feel the difference in how your lower-body muscles engage. Get out of the saddle and subtly shift your weight a bit forward and back, noting changes in weight and traction on each of your tires. Find that sweet spot.

DAY 5

Take a stand. As described in Chapter 3, sitting is the most efficient way to climb, but there are times when you need to stand, either for comfort or because the pitch is just too steep to stay seated. Out-of- the-saddle climbing is also a good exercise for strengthening your core and building fitness. Today, make it a point to practice standing climbing today. Deliberately stay up 10 to 20 pedal strokes past your usual comfort zone each time you do.

DAY 6

Shift early and often. We all know you're supposed to anticipate the shift (see page 32), but in reality, few of us—even those who have been at it a long time—practice it reliably on climbs. (I'm definitely guilty of just trying to muscle through a section rather than click my shifters. When I do the latter, it makes a huge difference in my ascent.) Today, focus your energy on using your shifters to stay in a comfortable (or as comfortable as possible on Day 6!) cadence. If there are sections you've been doing in your big ring, try them in your small ring to see if you're fresher at the top.

DAY 7

Practice pacing. Chances are good that you do not want to be on this freakin' hill today. You're likely at least a little tired physically, as well as mentally. So, today is a good day to practice pacing yourself. Roll onto the hill easier than planned and try to ride "negative splits," that is conserving enough energy through careful pacing to finish the climb a little stronger than when you started it.

DAY 8

Fuel up. As discussed in Chapter 8, eating to climb can be a sticky wicket. You need calories because climbing takes extra energy. Those calories are harder to digest because the hard work of pedaling against gravity diverts blood from your stomach into your muscles. Treat yourself today, and try a little candy to lift your spirits—and your legs. (Pros like Peter Sagan swear by gummy bears, and there was even a whole team sponsored by Jelly Belly jelly beans, which maybe uncoincidentally featured Phil Gaimon, one of the best climbers in the country.) Take in about 120 calories of your favorite fast-acting simple carbohydrate before today's climb, and see how you feel.

DAY 9

Time your breathing. You're at that point where you're getting close to the finish line but still too far out to smell the barn. Today is a good day to get a little Zen and work on clearing your mind and synchronizing your breathing to your pedal strokes. Try a rhythmic breathing technique, breathing in a five-count pattern when the hill is moderate and switching to a three-count pattern as it pitches upward. You'll be surprised at how the climb seems to go by more quickly and easily, even after all these times.

DAY 10

Go naked. Not literally, of course! But today, do the climb completely by feel. Turn your computer on, but put it in your pocket, or use your phone to record the ride. I guarantee that you'll notice something—a lawn gnome or some other cool yard art—you hadn't seen before in your previous nine trips up the hill. Soak in your surroundings, and really become one with the climb. You may like what you find.

DAY 11

Bring a friend. It's funny how pedaling in the company of others can change how you ride. Now that you've had a honeymoon phase with this climb, invite someone else to join you for the ascent. Notice how it changes your style and rhythm. Do you immediately ride faster right from the base? Are you slower or quicker to shift? Do you send yourself into the red more often? Make notes and try your best to climb your own climb, even in the company of others.

DAY 12

Up your self-talk game. Okay, you've got this. Today, you need to tell yourself that. Go full pro and use third person. "It's Day 12, Jaime. You *own* this climb." If a negative thought creeps in, drop it like a safe, and keep your positive mantras rolling smooth and steady and strong, just like you.

DAY 13

Work the other side. You've been going up—and down—the same climb. There's no doubt that you've gotten to know the descent pretty well and have probably consciously or subconsciously been implementing some of the techniques from Chapter 9. Today, don't think about the upside of the climb at all. Let it happen organically. Instead, focus on the downside and distributing your weight perfectly, for your most confident descent yet.

DAY 14

Pull it all together, and go for it. School's out! I know you're tired. I know you're not going into it properly recovered. But today is one of those days where you can really see the power of the mind, how even though you should be (and maybe are) cracked like a hard-boiled egg, you are capable of channeling the energy of your final push into a possible personal best. Pull together all the tips and techniques you've learned, pull out the stops, and see what happens. (Note: If you do crack and need to slow to a crawl, that's okay, too! You only find your limits when you reach them.)

(*REALLY*) ADVANCED CHALLENGE: "EVERESTING"

Obviously, you can't actually pedal your bike to the top of Mount Everest, the summit of which sits at the top of the world at 29,092 feet above sea level. But, you can get a pretty good idea of how hellish it would be, by "Everesting"—climbing the total height of Everest in a single ride. The feat has gained popularity in recent years and even has a website (everesting.cc) devoted to the endeavor, which includes a Hall of Fame for those who successfully do the deed.

The concept originated, interestingly enough, with George Mallory, grandson of the famous Everest climber of the same name. While training for his own Everest attempt, cycled up and down the 4,000-plus-foot Mount Donna Buang in Australia eight times in 1994. Nearly 20 years later, a band of climbing-obsessed Aussies, known as the Hells 500 crew, turned Everesting into a "thing," becoming the "creators and custodians" of the concept.

You can find all the fine print on their website, but the rules are pretty straightforward. You must climb 29,029 feet in a single ride, up and down

(continued on page 174)

↗ HELL, YES, I CLIMBED THAT!

THIS GRANDMOTHER CLIMBED ALPE D'HUEZ EIGHT TIMES IN ONE DAY!

Lori Hoechlin, 54, mother of four and grandmother of three,

an ultra-endurance cyclist from Rancho Mission Viejo, California, was sitting in a café eating breakfast in Orion, France, with a friend in 2015 when she announced that she "wanted to Everest." Her friend suggested Alpe d'Huez. Since they were only in town for a few days, Hoechlin didn't have much time to contemplate, so she jumped in with both feet and headed out to conquer the big climb the next morning.

Fellow *Bicycling* magazine contributor Jen See caught up with her to get the scoop on how it went, while we were gathering stories for this book. Here's what she told her.

"Coincidentally, the Tour [de France] was going through in a couple of days, and all the corners were already lined with fans. I had plenty to see. I went up and came back down. I went up again. People started recognizing me. By the sixth time, I was getting applause all the way up.

"I was in the Cycle Huez bike shop at the top of the climb to refuel about 9 hours in when I noticed that I was starting to get chafing from my bib shorts—they were wearing out! I bought myself another pair of Biemmes right there. It was also a good excuse to get a matching jersey. Then, I headed back out.

"My GPS watch lasts only 17 hours. All of a sudden, I felt it buzzing, and I saw 'low battery.' I was on my eighth and last lap. If my watch died, this wouldn't even count. I picked up the pace. In the Dutch corner, people filled the street, leaving me literally one narrow opening to ride through. They were clapping my back and blowing horns. It was so cold. I finally finished in 15 hours and 36 minutes, just before midnight. It was 134.1 miles.

"And, it actually wasn't a huge suffering. To me, it was just an extra-long day of doing something I love. I do double centuries. I've done RAAM. I sometimes think about what I could have done with racing if I'd started in my twenties or thirties. I don't regret it. It was worth it to invest in my kids for those years. But, I do wonder."

HOECHLIN'S EVERESTING TIPS

The details can make or break your Everest attempt. Hoechlin recommends having the following locked up before you set your sights on the eventual summit.

DIAL IN YOUR NUTRITION. Finding out what works for you nutrition-wise is huge. If you're properly fueling, you really don't feel any worse for wear at 12 hours in than you did at an hour in. You have to figure out what your body needs every hour. For me, I weigh around 120, and I take in around 200 to 250 calories per hour. That seems to keep me really steady.

BUILD A BASE CAMP. You definitely need to have a base camp somewhere. You have to have somewhere you put all your gear—your nutrition and hydration, your winter clothes, extra clothing.

CHARGE YOUR BATTERIES. Make sure that the lights are charged. Make sure that you have a way to keep your Garmin [or other GPS] unit charged. Some of the Garmin units don't last the time that it takes you to Everest, so you need to have some kind of external battery that you can plug into it. You want to make sure that you don't lose the tracking. That would be the worst.

BUILD YOUR ENDURANCE. If you're going to do 20,000 feet, you might as well go out and do an Everest. I'd just say, make sure that you're comfortable staying on the bike for 12-plus hours. You are going to have to do that. For some of these efforts, people are taking 22 to 24 hours.

PICK YOUR CLIMB. You want to pick something that's not so steep that it's going to chew up your legs, so that you can't get through it. To me, the right balance is somewhere right between 7- and 8-percent grade. I really want to find a straight, steady hill.

the same exact route, hill-repeat-style on one climb. You can take breaks to eat, but no sleeping. You'll also want to find a climb that gets as close to hitting the jackpot number as possible (not under obviously, but also not too far over) because only complete ascents count toward your goal, so if you hit the 29,029 halfway up your final ascent, you can't just call it good and turn around and cruise home. You need to finish the final ascent. The whole kit and caboodle needs to be tracked and submitted via a Strava file to get verified and for you to be accepted into the Hall of Fame.

Choosing the right route is of the essence for success. As my *Bicycling* magazine colleague Joe Lindsey noted in a piece he penned when Everesting burst on the scene a few years back, the ideal Everest climbs are "ones that feature an economy of miles to vertical, balanced against a climb that's repeatable." In other words, "Tackle a climb with a 19-percent wall and you'll knock out vertical quickly, but that eighth rep will kill you. Spread the gain over too long a distance, and nightfall is your nemesis; you'll be lucky to last as long as your Garmin battery."

To that end, he compiled this list of six great American climbs that hit this sweet spot. (Learn even more about a few of these iconic monsters in Chapter 11.)

MOUNT DIABLO, DANVILLE, CALIFORNIA

Length: 10.56 miles
Total ascent: 3,218.5 feet
Total ascents needed: 9
Total distance: 190 miles
The Strava page: strava.com/segments/mt-diablo-s-athenian-school-to-6806136

Used in several Tours of California, this San Francisco Bay Area summit finish has several routes to the top. The south side, from the Athenian

School, is ideal because it'll give you an Everesting in exactly nine ascents. That's the closest round number of ascents of any of our five candidates. But, you may want to descend a bit past the Athenian School each time—the margin of error here is mere meters, and if you come up short of 8,848, you will miss out.

PIKES PEAK, COLORADO SPRINGS, COLORADO

Length: 23.67 miles
Total ascent: 7,746 feet
Total ascents needed: 4
Total distance: 189.4 miles
The Strava page: strava.com/segments/pike-s-peak-625021

Sure, Mount Evans is taller. But Pikes Peak is far more suited to an Everest attempt: It's a shorter, steeper climb but still manageable. And, it's still a "14er," which is a massive Everesting ascent in the U.S.

MOUNT MITCHELL, BURNSVILLE, NORTH CAROLINA

Length: 4.7 miles
Total ascent: 1,381.2 feet
Total ascents needed: 21
Total distance: 197.4 miles
The Strava page: strava.com/segments/mount-mitchell-1546782

The centerpiece of the Blue Ridge classic ride, the Assault on Mount Mitchell, the highest peak in the eastern U.S. (6,684 feet) makes a great Everesting attempt. You'll need almost exactly 21 ascents (as with Diablo, start each lap a bit below the official Strava segment start to make sure you get to 8,848m), and while it's got some steep bits, there's also a less-nasty section in the middle that gives you some recovery.

(continued on page 178)

⊘ HELL, YES, I CLIMBED THAT!

THIS HILL JUNKIE DROPPED 70 POUNDS AND CRUSHED MOUNT WASHINGTON.

Doug Jansen, 55, of Pelham, New Hampshire, was 34 when an overweight, smoking, drinking colleague served him a wake-up call— literally—in the form of a slaying on the racquetball court.

"After my son was born, I changed jobs and stopped working out. Over about 10 years, I went from about 180 pounds to 230 pounds. The thing was, I thought of myself as 'stocky' but still fit. I wasn't.

"I got my butt handed to me. I couldn't volley the ball more than a few times before getting so winded and dizzy that I had to place both hands up against the wall and hang my head to catch my breath! I thought 'I'm going to die, if I don't get my health under control.'"

Despite the demoralizing circumstances, Jansen was hooked. He spent the next year riding regularly, cleaning up his diet, and shedding weight. Three years and 50 lost pounds later, he signed up for his first mountain bike race—Mount Snow, Vermont, not realizing how steep, up and down, the terrain would be. "I got my butt handed to me again," he recalls.

Back to the drawing board. Jansen sought training advice from his peers, who counseled him to get a road bike and work on endurance rides. He took to the pavement for long rides and left behind another 15 to 20 pounds. A year later, buoyed by his newfound trimness and fitness, he signed up for his first hill climb, the inaugural Ascutney climb in Mount Ascutney State Park in Vermont. Once again, he was surprised by what he found—2.5 miles that stayed at a torturous 15 percent for long stretches right off the line—but this time, he was prepared. He did well and was hooked for life.

"I did Mount Washington for the first time, too, that year, really having no idea how challenging 12 percent for 7.6 miles could be. I had a stock Specialized Allez with a triple crank. I was thinking if I could break 1:30, I'd be very happy." Jansen not only broke 1:30, he finished among the elites with a time of 1:14.

Jansen has since stood on many a podium and has put his tires to dirt in 48 states so far, missing only Louisiana and Mississippi. "I often go out of my way to find the most epic climbs an area has to offer, road or off-road. When others shuttle to a long descent, I ride. In Salida, Colorado, there's this ride called the Monarch Crest. The shuttle services will tell you the ride can only be done with a shuttle. BS! I've ridden up Highway 50 many times to make it a 54-mile loop. There are many other dirt routes up to the Crest that I've tried. I did meet a group of three one time that also was pedaling up to the Monarch Crest. One of the guys in that group (who also had done Mount Washington before) said climbing up to the Crest was the best part. Nearly brought a tear to my eye. So rare."

HALEAKALA, PAIA, HAWAII

Length: 34.5 miles
Total ascent: 9,711.3 feet
Total ascents needed: 3
Total distance: 207 miles
The Strava page: strava.com/segments/haleakala-%22world-s-longest-paved-climb%22-638944

You'll ride a monumental double century (plus!) to knock off this summit. What's more, you'll get long recovery stretches on each descent. Perhaps the best and worst part, simultaneously: Haleakala is a fairly steady climb. So, you can settle in on a good pace, but you have to pick that pace carefully, because there's no recovery.

ONION VALLEY ROAD, INDEPENDENCE, CALIFORNIA

Length: 4.5 miles
Total ascent: 2,457.4 feet
Total ascents needed: 12
Total distance: 108 miles
The Strava page: strava.com/segments/onion-valley-rd-climb-748107

This is the shortest distance route on the list. If successful, it would be one of the shortest on the Everesting Hall of Fame. But this segment of Onion Valley, in the remote Eastern Sierra Nevada of California, is a beast. It averages 10 percent over its 4.5-mile run, and the heat of an Owens Valley summer will beat you down. Start early.

MOUNT PALOMAR (SOUTH GRADE), PAUMA VALLEY, CALIFORNIA

Length: 11.6 miles
Total Ascent: 4,235.6 feet

Total ascents needed: 7
Total distance: 162.4 miles
The Strava page: strava.com/segments/palomar-mt-south-grade-taco-shop-to-273807

Yeah, sure—some guy named Chris Horner holds the Strava KOM for the fastest ascent of the south grade of Mount Palomar, arguably the top target for SoCal roadies. But, even Horner will bow to your magnificence after you climb it seven times in a day. Bonus: Jilberto's Taco Shop is at the bottom for all your refueling needs.

If you are particularly masochistic, you can try vEveresting, or virtual Everesting, which is as horrible as it sounds—completing the challenge virtually on an indoor trainer. The first self-flagellator to earn a vEveresting badge for this accomplishment was Frank Garcia, who pedaled 165 miles over 17 hours and 18 minutes, averaging a 7-percent grade in his rec room via his Wahoo Kickr smart trainer and Zwift (a virtual training program). Since Zwift is one big loop—a no-no in the Everesting universe—Garcia had to choose the program's one big climb—a 1,300-foot stretch called Watopia Wall—and ride up and down it a mind-blowing 314 times.

GET AFTER IT!

So long as you don't take the social fitness app Strava (see page 98) too seriously—and, seriously, please don't; people have died chasing downhill crowns—it's super-fun and can motivate you to dig that extra bit deeper on a climb, even when you're just riding solo.

Since this book is all about stepping up to various climbing challenges, I asked Strava Marketing Analyst Arjun Sudhir to curate the 20 longest Strava climbs in the U.S., as well as the 20 toughest to KOM/QOM. Turn the page, pick yours, and go for it. Note: In both lists, there are many duplicate or similar segments for a given general climb with slightly different start and end points. Where possible, preference was given to segments that had more total athlete activity attempts or views.

LONGEST CLIMBS, SORTED BY MILES

NAME	MILES	AVG. GRADE	FEET GAINED	LOCATION	STRAVA PAGE
Hilo to Mauna Kea	42.6	6.1	13,732	Hilo, HI	strava.com/segments/1504789
Haleakala Cycle to the Sun	35	5	9,921	Paia, HI	strava.com/segments/623325
Biggest KOM in the lower 48	32.3	6	9,976	Bishop, CA	strava.com/segments/10131042
El Paseo to Toro Peak	31.7	5.0	8,404	Palm Desert, CA	strava.com/segments/6940698
Three Rivers to Mineral King	26.0	5.0	6,880	Three Rivers, CA	strava.com/segments/10182589
East Fork–Dawson's Saddle	23.8	5.0	6,448	Azusa, CA	strava.com/segments/7734462
Pikes Peak	23.6	6.0	7,746	Manitou Springs, CO	strava.com/segments/625021
Dry Creek to Big Baldy through Whitaker Forest	23.6	5.0	6,283	Badger, CA	strava.com/segments/7193411
Lone Pine to Horseshoe Meadows via Tuttle Creek	22.3	5.0	6,219	Lone Pine, CA	strava.com/segments/12174627
Mt. Graham Full Monte–Paved	21.7	5.0	5,820	Safford, AZ	strava.com/segments/12213336

NAME	MILES	AVG. GRADE	FEET GAINED	LOCATION	STRAVA PAGE
Black Rock Rd. to Mckinley Grove Rd.—The back way to Wishon	21.7	5.0	5,816	Auberry, CA	strava.com/segments/12099301
SB Walmart to Keller Peak	21.4	6.0	7,895	Highland, CA	strava.com/segments/7429754
Grand Mesa (official full north side)	21	5.0	5,604	De Beque, CO	strava.com/segments/14979354
Bristlecone Climb to visitors center	20.8	6.0	6,174	Big Pine, CA	strava.com/segments/12856385
Bottom to lookout via Squaw Creek Rd.	20.7	6.0	6,623	Riggins, ID	strava.com/segments/8079031
Coho to Summit via S. Lincoln & E. 8th	19.6	5.0	5,244	Port Angeles, WA	strava.com/segments/12856736
South Lake Climb—McLaren to South Lake parking lot	19.3	5.0	5,435	Bishop, CA	strava.com/segments/5678081
The Whole Tostada	19.3	5.3	5,442	Moab, UT	strava.com/segments/13338185
The Big Sequoia	19.2	5.0	5,399	Three Rivers, CA	strava.com/segments/3669536
Lee Canyon full climb to ski lodge	17.1	6.0	5,290	Las Vegas, NV	strava.com/segments/734755

TOUGHEST TO KOM, SORTED BY FEET GAIN

NAME	MILES	AVG GRADE	FEET GAINED	LOCATION	STRAVA PAGE
Full Ascent from Saddle Road to the top	15.0	9.0	7,184	Mauna Kea Forest Reserve, HI	strava.com/segments/3040497
Mt. Washington*	7.3	12.0	4,685	Gorham, NH	strava.com/segments/3237
Black Bear Road Climb	6.7	11.0	3,797	Telluride, CO	strava.com/segments/7641107
Empire to End of Guardsman	8.5	9.0	3,903	Park City, UT	strava.com/segments/10596725
GT—Aspen Mountain Hill Climb	4.6	13.0	3,193	Aspen, CO	strava.com/segments/10428297
Barr Trail to Heizer turnoff	4.5	12.0	2,789	Monument, CO	strava.com/segments/829961
Gridley Trailhead to Nordoff Lookout Tower	6.9	9.0	3,335	Ojai, CA	strava.com/segments/840104
Powder Mountain Hill Climb	6.0	10.0	3,106	Eden, UT	strava.com/segments/671261
Sun Top Fire Road Climb	5.8	10.0	3,020	Enumclaw, WA	strava.com/segments/613628
Copper Mountain-Colorado Trail to top of Wheeler Pass	3.7	13.0	2,639	Frisco, CO	strava.com/segments/2102671

*Can only get this one through the official Mount Washington Hillclimb race, I'm afraid—the road is closed to bicycles the rest of the year.

NAME	MILES	AVG GRADE	FEET GAINED	LOCATION	STRAVA PAGE
4 miles up mag	3.8	10.0	2,004	Nederland, CO	strava.com/segments/1466351
La Porte Climb	5.7	8.0	2,494	Plumas County, CA	strava.com/segments/4235021
Soda Springs v2	5.3	8.0	2,368	Los Gatos, CA	strava.com/segments/9583505
Nate Harrison Grade: Top Half	5.2	8.0	2,301	Pauma Valley, CA	strava.com/segments/3630070
Calistoga to Holms	4.4	8.0	2,301	Calistoga, CA	strava.com/segments/9700896
Race to the top of Vermont	4.1	11.0	2,437	Stowe, VT	strava.com/segments/735766
Ranger to Ski Lift Driveway	4.6	8.0	2,081	Mount Baldy, CA	strava.com/segments/3349968
Bean Mountain full climb	3.7	12.0	2,304	Delano, TN	strava.com/segments/11344701
Trabuco Trail (Up)	3.8	11.0	2,165	Corona, CA	strava.com/segments/777533
SBT: 1st 3.3 miles up (Taos to tree drop)	3.3	12.0	2,052	Taos, NM	strava.com/segments/4239779

REFERENCES

CHAPTER 1

E. Morita, et al. "Psychological effects of forest environments on healthy adults: Shinrin-yoku (forest-air bathing, walking) as a possible method of stress reduction. *Public Health*, 121, no. 1 (2007 Jan): 54–63. Epub 2006 Oct 20.

Mark J. Nieuwenhujsen, et al. "Positive health effects of the natural outdoor environment in typical populations in different regions in Europe (PHENOTYPE): a study programme protocol." *BMJ*, 4, no. 2 (2014): e004951.

Seresinhe, C. I., et al. "Quantifying the impact of scenic environments on health."

Scientific Reports, 5, 16899 (2015). doi: 10.1038/srep16899 (2015).

Richard M. Ryan, et al. "Vitalizing effects of being outdoors and in nature." *Journal of Environmental Psychology*, 30, no. 2 (June 2010): 159–68.

American Chemical Society. "Green space can make people happier for years." Environmental Science and Technology, *January 8, 2014.*

CHAPTER 2

Michael Hutchinson. "What can we learn from Chris Froome's power data?" July 21, 2015. cyclingweekly.com/news/racing/tour-de-france/what-can-we-learn-from-chris-froomes-power-data-183677.

CHAPTER 5

B. R. Ronnestad. "Strength training improves performance and pedaling characteristics in elite cyclists." *Scandinavian Journal of Medicine and Science in Sports,* 25, no. 1 (Feb 2015): e89–98. doi: 10.1111/sms.12257.

K. Beattie, et al. "The effect of maximal- and explosive-strength training on performance indicators in cyclists." *International Journal of Sports Physiology and Performance,* 12, no. 4 (April 2017): 470–80.

A. Sunde, et al. "Maximal strength training improves cycling economy in competitive cyclists." *Journal of Strength and Conditioning Research,* 24, no. 8 (2010 Aug): 2157–65. doi: 10.1519/JSC.0b013e3181aeb16a.

O. Vikmoene, et al. "Heavy strength training improves running and cycling performance following prolonged submaximal work in well-trained female athletes." *Physiological Reports,* 5, no. 5 (2017 March): e13149. doi: 10.14814/phy2.13149.

Paul B. Laursen, et al. "Interval training program optimization in highly trained endurance cyclists." *Medicine and Science in Sports and Exercise,* 34, no. 11 (2002 Nov): 1801–7.

C. D. Paton and W. G. Hopkins. "Combining explosive and high-resistance training improves performance in competitive cyclists." *Journal of Strength and Conditioning Research,* 19, no. 4 (2005 Nov): 826–30.

CHAPTER 6

T. D. Noakes. "Fatigue is a brain-derived emotion that regulates the exercise behavior to ensure the protection of whole-body homeostasis." *Frontiers in Physiology,* 3, no. 82 (2012 April 11): doi: 10.3389/fphys.2012.00082.

S. M. Marcora, et al. "Mental fatigue impairs physical performance in humans." *Journal of Applied Physiology,* 106, no. 3 (2009 March): 857–64. doi: 10.1152/japplphysiol.91324.2008.

C. R. Abbiss and P. B. Laursen. "Models to explain fatigue during prolonged endurance cycling." *Sports Medicine,* 35, no. 10 (2005): 865–98.

Karen Van Proeyen, et al. "Beneficial metabolic adaptations due to endurance exercise training in the fasted state." *Journal of Applied Physiology,* 110, no. 1: 236–45. doi: 10.1152/japplphysiol.00907.2010.

H. Rauch, et al. "A signalling role for muscle glycogen in the regulation of pace during prolonged exercise." *British Journal of Sports Medicine,* 39, no. 1 (2005 Jan): 34–38.

CHAPTER 8

Consumer Reports: Body-Fat Scale Review (March 11, 2016): consumerreports.org/body-fat-scales/body-fat-scale-review/

G. Pounis, et al. "Association of pasta consumption with body mass index and waist-to-hip ratio: results from Moli-sani and INHES studies." *Nutrition & Diabetes,* 6 (2016): e218. doi:10.1038/nutd.2016.20.

Justin McCarthy. "Americans not avoiding fat and salt as much." July 27, 2015. news.gallup.com/poll/184340/americans-not-avoiding-fat-salt.aspx.

L. J. van Loon. "Is there a need for protein ingestion during exercise?" *Sports Medicine,* 44, suppl 1: S105–11. doi: 10.1007/s40279-014-0156-z.

Yung-Chih Chen, et al. "Feeding influences adipose tissue responses to exercise in overweight men. *American Journal of Physiology—Endocrinology and Metabolism* (2017): doi: 10.1152/ajpendo.00006.2017.

CHAPTER 11

Nicholas Bakalar. "High altitudes may aid weight control." April 23, 2014. well.blogs.nytimes.com/2014/04/23/high-altitudes-may-aid-weight-control/?_r=0

Marco Zaccaria, et al. "Decreased serum leptin levels during prolonged high altitude exposure." *European Journal of Applied Science*, 92, no. 3 (July 2004): 249–53. doi.org/10.1007/s00421-004-1070-0.

INDEX

Boldface page references indicate photographs and *italic* page references indicate sidebars and tables.

A
ABSA Cape Epic, xii
Adenosine, 82
Adenosine triphosphate (ATP), 127
Adirondacks, 147
Aerobic metabolism, 75
Air resistance, 13, 14
Alcohol, 106
Allen, Hunter, 9, 34
Altitude, 20, 144. *See also* high altitude
AMGEN Tour of California, 99
Anabolic state, 71
Applegate, Andy, 83, 116
ATP. *See* adenosine triphosphate

B
Ball pike (exercise), 54, **54**
Barbells, 62, **62**
Barton, Eric, 128
Base, 37, 38–39
Base-building rides, 41
Base training, 38–43
Belichick, Bill, 80

Bicycling, 90, 132
Big climbs. *See also* "Everesting"
   climbing for, 152–56
   Le Mauna Kea as, 142–43
   Mount Baldy as, 145–46
   Mount Evans as, 143–44
   Mount Mitchell as, 150
   Mount Washington as, 151–52
   Onion Valley as, 146–47
   Pikes Peak as, 148–49
Big gear acceleration, 69
Bikes, 13–14, 27, 98, 122
Black Mountains, 150
Blood plasma levels, 77
Body, 46–47, 77
   arms of, 29, 30
   categories for, 25
   during crests, 36
   mind separate from, 11
   during pedaling, 28
   positioning of, 168
   relaxation of, 83
Body types, 22
Body weight, 24–27, 100–104

Bonci, Leslie, 106
Box jumps, 65, **65**, 70
Brain
   climbing influence on, 6
   glucose for, 82
   hilly rides and, 127
   oxygen for, 153
Brakes, 117, 119
Breathing, 73
   heavy huffing during, 34
   motivation with, 81
   oxygen with, 153
   pacing with, 139
   with pedal stroke, 82, 170
   timing of, 169
Breck Epic, 152
Bridge (exercise), 52, **52**

C

Cadence, 30–32, 168
Calories, 102. *See also* empty calories
Canaan Valley Resort, xi–xii
Cannabinoids, 6
Carbohydrates, 106, 108–9
Cassettes, 91, 93
Catabolic state, 71
Center of mass, 16
Chain friction, 13–14
Chainrings, 91, 92, 93
Circulatory system, 4
Climb categories, 21
Climb challenges, 167–79
Climbing intervals, 45
Climb plan, 158–59, **158–59**, 160–63, **160–63**
Climbs. *See also* big climbs
   altitude during, 143
   eating for, 112
   with endurance, 33
   fuel for, 83
   gears and, 89
   Haleakala as, 142
   motivation for, 80
   pitch of, 78
   seated climb in, 28–29
   steep climbs in, 36, 146
Coasting, 17
Coates, Budd, 82
Cobra lift (exercise), 50, **50**
Cognitive fatigue, 11
Colorado Rockies, 2, 143
Colorado Springs, 148
Columbine racecourse, 1–2

Connective tissue, 60
Contador, Alberto, 24
Contrast shower, 72
Core, 5–6
Core body temperature, 77
Core training
   ball pike for, 54, **54**
   bridge for, 52, **52**
   building of, 46–47
   cobra lift for, 50, **50**
   on-bike for, 55
   Russian twist for, 53, **53**
   scorpion for, 51, **51**
   TT plank, 49, **49**
Crankset, 92
Crashes, 120
Cravens, Sherman, 85
Crests, 36
Criterium rider, 9
Crystal Reservoir Visitor Center, 149
Curves, 119
Cycle to the Sun, 143
Cycling
   dress code for, 96, 97
   physics for, 13
   with power-to-weight ratio, 24
   with seated climb, 28–29
Cycling Today, 21
Cyclist's Training Bible, The (Friel), 24

D

Davenport, Paul W., 5
Deadlifts, 62, **62**
Deep breathing, 73
Dehydration, 155
Descents, 115–19, 120, 121, 122
Diets, 2
   alcohol in, 106
   gut microbiomes and, 105
   incarnations of, 104
   protein in, 107
Di Savino, Victoria, 27, 85
Dombrowski, Joe, 146
Drivetrain, 91
Dumbbells, 61, **61**

E

Ectomorph, 25, 27
Efficiency, 58–59
Empty calories, 105–6
Endomorph, 25, 27–28
Endorphins, 6

Endurance, 67, 166, 172, 176
   in base training, 38, 39
   building of, 173
   climbing with, 33, 165
   fatigue and, 75
   for legs, 76
"Everesting," 171–79. *See also* virtual Everesting
Exercise
   box jumps in, 65, **65**
   cobra life as, 50, **50**
   deadlifts in, 62, **62**
   intervals in, 67–70
   leg presses in, 63, **63**
   plank position as, 54, **54**
   squats in, 61, **61**
   stronger muscles with, 59
   weighted jump squats in, 66, **66**
   weights in, 59–60
Explosive lifting, 64
Extended burst, 45

F

Fajans, Joel, 13, 16
Fasted training, 78, 112–13
Fasting, 111–13
Fast-twitch muscle fiber, 40, 58
Fat, 107, 108
Fatigue, 11
Fleshner, Monika R., 6
Force production, 64
Ford, Henry, 79
Frame (body), 46–47
Freak-out flowchart, 76
Frenemies, 3
Friel, Joe, 24
Froome, Chris, 15
FTP. *See* functional threshold power
Fuel, 169. *See also* oxygen
   body weight and, 100
   carbohydrates as, 108–9
   for climbs, 83
   hydration and, 79
   with recovery, 109–10
Full-recovery full throttles, 68
Functional threshold power (FTP), 126

G

Gaimon, Phil, 146
Gearing, 90–91, 92
Gear rationales, 91–94
Gear ratios, 91–94

Gears
   cadence maintained with, 32
   with chain friction, 13–14
   climbing and, 89
   gradient and, 90
   hills and, 130
   for steep climbs, 36
Giddings, Caitlin, 7
Glucose, 82
Glutes, 48
Glycogen, 75, 77, 78, 103, 127
Goat Hill, 18, 19
Grades, 1–2, 17, 19–20, 144, 149
Gradient, 18–19, 90
Grand Tour, 95
Gran Fondos, 95
Graves, Mark, 85
Griffin, Dina, 71
Ground contact, 95
Gut microbiomes, 105

H

Haleakala, 142, 178
Hamilton, Tyler, 148
Heart, 4
Heart rate, 26, 38, 43, 130
   cadence in, 31
   with high altitude, 153–54
   with pace, 45
   power proportional with, 14
High altitude, 153–54, 155
High-intensity interval training (HIIT), 41, 67
High-resistance training, 64
HIIT. *See* high-intensity interval training
Hillary, Edmund, 10
Hill charges, 68
Hill climbs, 136–37
Hills, 6, 18
   big climbs with, 151
   difficultly for, 19–20
   gears and, 130
   for legs, 4
   power for, 15
   steepness on, 17
   success for, 34
   training for, 128–30
   training without, 46
Hilly rides, 126–31
Hips, 48, **48**, 51, **51**
Hoechlin, Lori, 172, 173
Horner, Chris, 179
Hors Catégorie, 21

Hungry, 110
Hurford, Molly, 132
Hydration, 79, 99

I

Ice bath, 71–72
Inclines, 14, 18–19
Intervals, 135, 158, *158*. *See also* tolerance intervals
    base training and, 42–43
    in exercises, 67–70
    improvement of, 78
    LT in, 43, 45
    stage for, 138–39

J

Jansen, Doug, 142, *176*, *177*

K

Keener, Jeff, *129*
Klausutis, T. J., 1, 2, 3, 6, 21–22
Kona Endurance and Adventure Team, 64

L

Lactate, 40, 75
Lactate threshold (LT), 6, 86, *166*
    in base training, 39
    field test for, 44
    in intervals, 43, 45
    muscles and, 67
    power and, 32
    strong base for, 37
Laursen, Paul, 41, 67
Leadville racecourse, 1
Lee, Michelle, 122
Legs
    cadence for, 30, 31
    endurance for, 76
    metabolic magic for, 3–4
    presses for, 63, **63**
    with repeats, 131
    sliding and, 86
Light, natural, 11
Lightning danger, 150
Lim, Allen, 126
Lindsey, Joe, *174*
Liver, 77
Long, steady climbs, 36
Longest climbs, by miles, 180–83

LT. *See* lactate threshold
Lungs, 5

M

Mallory, George, 141, *171*
Marling, Ian, *84*
Masters Nationals Road race, 9
Match-burning, 35
Mauna Kea, 142–43
Maximum heart rate (MHR), 38
MCT-4, 41
Medicine ball, 53, **53**
Mental training, 6, 9
Mesomorph, 25, 28
Metabolic flexibility, 78
Metabolic magic, 3–6, 40, 72
Metabolic waste, 70
Metrics, 33
MHR. *See* maximum heart rate
Mind, 11, 58, 79
Mitochondria, 4–5
Mitochondrial lactate oxidation complex (mLOC), 41
Mood-lifter, 6, 11
Motivation, 80–81. *See also* positive thoughts
Mountain bikes, xi–xii, *93*, *95*
Mountainside, *84*
Mount Baldy, 145–46
Mount Diabol, *174*
Mount Evans, 143–44
Mount Everest, 10
Mount Kilimanjaro, 5
Mount Lemmon, 144–45
Mount Mitchell, 150, *175*
Mount Palomar, *178*
Mount Ventoux, 16
Mount Washington, 151–52, *177*
Mount Washington Auto Road Bicycle Hillclimb, 24, 89
Mozaffarian, Dariush, 107
Muscle-fiber, 57, 105, 127, 135
Muscles. *See also* core
    anabolic state and, 71
    cadence with, 31
    development of, 59–60
    electrical stimulation for, 73
    for endomorph, 27–28
    exercise for stronger, 59
    glycogen in, 75
    on inclines, 19
    inflammation in, 103
    LT and, 67

mind connection to, 58
recovery for, 70

N
Nutrition, 104–11, 173

O
Onion Valley, 146–47, 178
On-the-bike speed, 67
Oxygen
    altitude for less, 20
    in base training, 40
    during big climbs, 152
    for brain, 153
    at Mauna Kea, 142
    mitochondria delivered by, 4–5

P
Pacing, 45, 139–40, 169
Patience, 7–10
Peaks Coaching Group, 8, 9, 27, 34
Pedaling, 28–31
Pedal stroke, 17–18
    breathing with, 82, 170
    physics of, 97
    power in, 24–28
Pennsylvania Perimeter Ride Against Cancer (PPRAC), 86
Pennsylvania racecourse, 34
Persistence, 7–10
Physics, 13, 15, 21–22
Pikes Peak, 148–50, 175
Plank position (exercise), 54, **54**
Plyometrics, 64, 65, **65**, 66, **66**
Positive thoughts, 81
Post-exercise, 71
Pounds per square inch (psi), 94
Pounds-to-inches, 26
Power, 126
    altitude decline of, 154
    for grades, 17
    hardness of, 32–33
    heart rate proportional to, 14
    for hills, 15
    in pedal stroke, 24–28
    standing pedaling for, 29
    steepness and, 16
    strength training of, 57
Power Mountain, 151
Power position, 83
Power surges, 69

Power-to-weight, 23–26, 57, 104
PPRAC. *See* Pennsylvania Perimeter Ride Against Cancer
Protein, 107, 109
Psi. *See* pounds per square inch
Punchy ups, 68

Q
Qigong climbing, 83

R
Races, xi–xii, 3, 9, 24
Racioppi, Anne, 10
Ramps, 69–70
Recovery, 68, 158, 158, 166
    flushes for, 140
    replenish fuel with, 109–10
    right way to, 70–73
Relaxation techniques, 73
Repeats
    for "Everesting," 174
    legs with, 131
    performance of, 121–23
    rocket drills as, 135
    rock the rollers as, 134
Rewards, xii–xiii
Riders, 3, 16, 23, 24
Riding uphill, xiii
Road conditions, 20
Rock the rollers, 33, 36
Rolling resistance, 13–14
Runner's World Running on Air (Coates), 82
Rusch, Rebecca, 5, 71
Russian twist (exercise), 53, **53**

S
Saddlebags, 98
Sagan, Peter, 115, 146
Saint Kevin, 1
Salamander Slope, xi–xii
San Millán, Iñigo, 41
Scenic environments, 11
Scheske, Todd, 8, 27
Scorpion (exercise), 51, **51**
Scrub speeding, 117
Seated climb, 28–29
See, Jen, 172
Serotonin, 82
Shea, Marti, 25, 90
Shirley, Neil, 146, 147

Sierra Nevada, 146
Simmons, Jonathan, 85
Sims, Stacy, 102
Sleep, 72, 103, 110
Sliding, 86
Slow-twitch muscle fibers, 39, 40
Smart bikes, 91
Speed, 17, 25, 118
Spence, Evelyn, 136
Sprinter's climb, 33, 36
Sprinting, 8, 9
Squats, 61, **61**
Stability ball, 54, **54**
Stage race, 152. *See also* Breck Epic
Stage races, 131
Standing pedaling, 29, 30
Steep climbs, 36, 146
Steepest grade, 19
Steep hills, 132–33
Steepness, 16, 17. *See also* grades
Strava, 15, 24, 98, 174
Strength training, 57, 58–59
Stress, 6
Sudhir, Arjun, 179
Sugarloaf Pass, 1
Sumner, Jason, 149
Super-compensation mode, 103
Switchbacks, 64
System flush, 73

T

Tabata, Izumi, 67
Tabata intervals, 67
Taper, 110, 111
Thermoregulation system, 78
Thompson, Dylan, 111
Thornton, Tommy, 116
Time trial (TT), 80
Tipping bird, 48, **48**
Tires, 94, 95
Tolerance intervals, 44–45
Torso, 29, 30
Tour de France, 15, 21
Tour de Garage, 130
Tour of California, 145
Track racing, 8
Training, 2, 8, 33, 157–58, 166, 176. *See also* mental training

Training and Racing with Power Meter (Allen), 34
TT. *See* time trial
TT plank (exercise), 49, **49**
Turner, Glenn, 28
12 week climb plan, 160, 161, 162
24 Hours of Canaan, xi–xii

U

Ultra-endurance cyclist, 172
Uphill coasting, 17
Uphill riding, 64

V

Vaughan, Brian, 99
Verheul, John, 108, 110
Vertical distance, 21
Virtual Everesting, 179

W

Warm ups, 64, 67
Waschusett Mountain, 8
Watts
   in body weight, 26
   for cyclists, 16
   for hilly rides, 126
   power as, 15
   speed with, 17
Weight, 104, 168
Weighted jump squats, 66, **66**
Weight loss, 177
   glycogen in, 103
   pacing for, 110
   plans for, 101, 102, 104
Weights, 59–60
Werner, Kerry, 64
Wheel rotation, 96
Whiteface Mountain, 147–48
Willet, Kirk, 148

Z

Zones
   base with, 38–39
   blending of, 43
   in training, 166